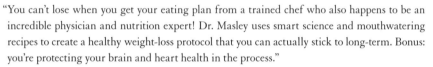

"You can't lose when you get your eating plan from a trained chef who also happens to be an incredible physician and nutrition expert! Dr. Masley uses smart science and mouthwatering recipes to create a healthy weight-loss protocol that you can actually stick to long-term. Bonus: you're protecting your brain and heart health in the process."
—**JJ VIRGIN, *New York Times* bestselling author of *The Virgin Diet* and *The Sugar Impact Diet***

"Leveraging the very best in nutritional science, Dr. Masley has truly created the Mediterranean diet '2.0' and skillfully guides the reader through its implementation."
—**DAVID PERLMUTTER, MD, *New York Times* bestselling author of *Grain Brain* and *Brain Wash***

"If you want to protect your heart, brain, and gut health all while losing weight, this is the book for you. The program detailed in this innovative book is easy to follow and—most important—deliciously satisfying."
—**DANIEL G. AMEN, MD, founder of the Amen Clinics and *New York Times* bestselling author of *Change Your Brain, Change Your Life***

"Combines traditional Mediterranean wisdom with the very latest in nutritional science to create a way of eating that's fresh, delicious, slimming, and *incredibly* good for you. This is a plan you can follow—and love—for life."
—**KELLYANN PETRUCCI, MS, ND, *New York Times* bestselling author of *Dr. Kellyann's Bone Broth Diet***

"There are arguably no diets backed by as much powerful evidence as the Mediterranean diet. Likewise there are also fewer if any experts better poised to guide you through the Mediterranean diet than Dr. Steven Masley. Almost anyone could do well by adopting his advice."
—**ALAN CHRISTIANSON, NMD, *New York Times* bestselling author of *The Adrenal Reset Diet* and *The Metabolism Reset Diet***

"We all need to get back to what has worked for the Mediterranean peoples for centuries. This book is a great place to start and a genuine must-read! It's a superb, comprehensive, and easy-to-read book on nutritional healing."
—**STEPHEN T. SINATRA, MD, bestselling author of *The Sinatra Solution***

"Dr. Masley makes eating well easy and enjoyable. My favorite 'Method' recipe is one you might not associate with Mediterranean cuisine: the breakfast shake. It's a phenomenally delicious and nutritious way to start the day. You'll be able to find the ingredients of his plan anywhere, and with his clear explanations and authoritative instructions, he'll make you feel like a gourmet chef!"

—ROBYN OPENSHAW, MSW, LCSW, founder of GreenSmoothieGirl.com, bestselling author of *Vibe* and *The Green Smoothies Diet*

"What do you get when you cross a world-renowned physician/nutritionist with a trained gourmet chef? You get Dr. Steven Masley! In this absolutely wonderful book, Dr. Masley presents a novel way of eating that puts a low-glycemic twist on the Mediterranean diet. You'll never miss the sugar, and the recipes are fantastic!"

—JONNY BOWDEN, PhD, CNS, board-certified nutritionist, bestselling author of *The 150 Healthiest Foods on Earth*

"The next best thing to actually living there, *The Mediterranean Method* gives you all of the flavors and ingredients of the healthiest region in the world but none of the deprivation you might associate with a 'diet.' Dr. Masley is an expert clinician, physician, and foodie, ensuring that his plan will deliciously improve the lives of all!"

—ANNA CABECA, DO, author of *The Hormone Fix*

"If you're looking for a delicious way to eat without all the diet jargon and special ingredients, this is your book. Dr. Masley is brilliant—he explains the science behind the Mediterranean eating style but also gives you delicious, flavorful, and simple recipes for adopting this healthful way of life. He's also a real chef—I've cooked with him and know he's the best. I highly, highly recommend this book!"

—LEANNE ELY, author of *Saving Dinner*

"Dr. Masley provides the best explanation and application yet of this famous dietary and lifestyle approach. . . . I recommend it with enthusiasm."

—DALE E. BREDESEN, MD, founding president and professor emeritus of the Buck Institute for Research on Aging, author of *The End of Alzheimer's*

"Because he's a doctor, Steven Masley's protocol will help you lose weight, protect your heart and brain, and live longer. Because he's also a trained chef, his mouthwatering *Mediterranean Method* recipes will make you hugely popular around the family table!"

—ANTHONY YOUN, MD, America's Holistic Plastic Surgeon, author of *The Age Fix*

"Dr. Steven Masley is a brilliant, holistic, functional medicine practitioner who has been teaching doctors and patients for more than thirty years, and his passion for food is so deep that he's professionally trained as a chef. *The Mediterranean Method* is his brilliant, modern update on an ancient diet. The recipes are simple yet elegant—and delicious. The book is destined to be dog-eared as you successfully try these recipes again and again."

—TOM O'BRYAN, DC, CCN, DACBN, author of *You Can Fix Your Brain*

The Mediterranean Method

*Your Complete Plan to
Harness the Power of the
Healthiest Diet on the Planet—
Lose Weight,
Prevent Heart Disease,
and More!*

Steven Masley, MD

HARMONY BOOKS
NEW YORK

Also by Steven Masley, MD

Ten Years Younger

The 30-Day Heart Tune-Up

Smart Fat (with coauthor Jonny Bowden)

The Better Brain Solution

Copyright © 2019 by Steven Masley, MD
Photographs copyright © 2019 by Robert Bredvad

All rights reserved.
Published in the United States by Harmony Books, an imprint of Random House, a division of Penguin Random House LLC, New York. harmonybooks.com

Harmony Books is a registered trademark, and the Circle colophon is a trademark of Penguin Random House LLC.

Originally published in hardcover in the United States by Harmony Books, an imprint of the Crown Publishing Group, a division of Penguin Random House LLC, New York, in 2019.

Library of Congress Cataloging-in-Publication Data is available.

ISBN 978-0-593-13637-9
Ebook ISBN 978-0-593-13604-1

Printed in the United States of America

Book and cover design by Jan Derevjanik
Photographs by Robert Bredvad

3rd Printing

First Paperback Edition

To Nicole for her ongoing love and support

Contents

INTRODUCTION

The world-famous Mediterranean diet is based upon the eating habits of people living around the Mediterranean Sea. It has an almost unlimited diversity of fresh and delicious foods. Technically, it is not a "diet" at all but, rather, it reflects the culinary traditions of varied countries on at least three continents—not just Italy, France, and Spain but also Greece, Turkey, Israel, Lebanon, Syria, Egypt, Morocco, Tunisia, and more.

What these cuisines have in common is the consumption of a variety of fresh, seasonal whole foods. More specifically, the Mediterranean diet features an abundance of vegetables, fruits, beans, nuts, herbs, and spices; moderate amounts of seafood and poultry; the use of extra-virgin olive oil instead of butter and unhealthy fats; and with meals, moderate consumption of red wine (in most regions). When Mediterranean peoples eat grains, they traditionally reach for whole grains such as barley, millet, farro, wheat berries, or bulgur.

What the Mediterranean diet has avoided is processed foods, sugar, artificial flavors, refined flour, and unhealthy fats. Red meats are rarely on the menu or are used sparingly to flavor a dish. In contrast to crazy fad diets that tell you what *not* to eat, this diet focuses on the right foods to *add*, saving treats for special occasions. Those trendy diets come and go, but the time-tested Mediterranean eating plan has been around for thousands of years.

The diverse and flavorful foods are wonderful—but there is another plus to the Mediterranean diet. It is the best diet for your health, and in polls like *U.S. News & World Report*'s annual diet roundup, it consistently ranks as the #1 diet on the planet, as rated by nutritionists, researchers, doctors, and other health-care experts. To wit: Native Mediterranean dwellers have some of the longest life spans ever recorded, living—disease free—into their 80s, 90s, and beyond. They are slimmer and have less obesity. They have lower rates for heart disease, memory loss, and cancer. The people of Spain, who tend to follow the Mediterranean diet closely, have the longest life span and the best health of those in any country in the Western world.

Here's another reason that the Mediterranean way of eating gets so many votes as the world's best all-around diet: It's very easy to follow. Recipes are fun and easy to prepare, and your family and friends will love the meals that you'll serve.

This brings me to why I have chosen to write this book. For decades, I've worked as a physician-researcher, nutritionist, and author, and I have been committed to guiding patients in my clinic (as well as my readers) toward a healthier, happier lifestyle that benefits both mind and body—one free of chronic illness, pain, and preventable diseases, from cardiovascular disease to diabetes, from cancer to memory loss, Alzheimer's, and so much more. Many know me as a doctor who integrates the foundations of everyday nutrition, physical activity, and informed lifestyle choices as the keys to achieving optimum wellness and longevity. But few know that I'm as devoted to great-tasting food as I am to great health. Being able to bring you the Mediterranean diet is a dream come true—a perfect combination of two passions that happen to be both personal and professional.

Many years ago, as I was on the brink of entering into a particularly intense phase of my medical training, the Mediterranean way of eating—as well as the whole lifestyle away from the table—captured my attention.

Though I was preparing to begin medical school, I felt a strong urge to put my studies on hold and go see the world before I buckled down and focused on my future medical career. I knew that breaking out of my familiar academic and hospital environments and meeting a range of new people would ultimately make me a better doctor—one who would be more capable of relating to a variety of patients. With $150 in my pocket, some classroom French, and a meager list of contacts, I found myself in the South of France, looking for work. I landed upon it in the seaside city of Cannes, captaining a boat for an American banker who also hired me to cook for him and his guests. I was a fairly experienced sailor, but though I loved cooking and was pretty good at it, my chef's skills were still a work in progress and I'd be cooking in a small galley kitchen. Fortunately, my new boss gave me carte blanche to source ingredients for meals from some of the best markets and food shops on earth.

In the bustling old port in Cannes, as well as several tiny, humble villages dotting the region, I shopped each day for fresh seafood plucked from the water not more than one day before; an endless variety of vegetables grown with nothing but sunshine, rain, and rich soil; generous bunches of herbs that smelled like summer; and perfectly ripened fruits bursting with flavors I'd never tasted. I chose from an array of handmade cheeses, nuts, dried beans, oils and vinegars, spices and mustards, farm-fresh eggs, creamy yogurt, a smattering of poultry and pasture-raised meats, exquisite chocolates, and freshly baked breads. Plus, there were wine shops featuring wines from every region in France, as well as other parts of Europe.

Everything I wanted to cook and serve was in port, at a centuries-old market, in a family-run corner shop or a vendor's stall, sometimes sold by the person who'd made, grown, or gathered the item. Unlike how our grocery stores are stocked in the United States, with processed and pre-pared foods loaded with shelf-stabilizing preservatives or out-of-season oddities, the local attitude seemed to be that if it wasn't available that day, then it wasn't worth eating. The in-season real foods I put in my market basket—foundations of the true Mediterranean diet—changed my life.

Of course, I would learn it wasn't just France. From travels along the coasts of Italy, Spain, and Greece and on islands like Corsica, Sardinia, Sicily, and Crete, I dis-covered that this fresh, wholesome food was abundant; and after travel farther afield in countries like Turkey, Morocco, Egypt, and across North Africa, as well as Portugal to the west and Middle Eastern countries to the east, just beyond the Mediterranean basin, the influence of these regional ingredients made for cuisines that overlapped and had much in common—and not just olive oil.

I was hooked on the food—I even did a stint cooking in a French restaurant before I returned to the United States—and I wanted to eat like that all the time. As a physician I would eventually learn that doing so was the healthiest choice a person could make, but it took me a while to reach that conclusion.

Once I reached medical school, the pre-vailing medical wisdom and my medical colleagues led me to follow and recommend a fairly strict, low-fat eating plan, including popular programs at the time that largely ignored healthy fats, generous portions of vegetables, fruits, beans, and clean proteins. We believed that such a rigid diet prescrip-tion was the best choice for heart health, even

as rates of obesity and diabetes continued to climb.

After a decade in clinical practice, I started performing randomized dietary interventions to help patients who wanted to lose weight and get healthy. I initially offered a diet that was popular in the media at the time, the Ornish program, which was vegetarian and ultra-low in fat. Even though cardiologist Dr. Dean Ornish had published results showing a slight reversal in heart disease, something unheard of at the time, the problem was that 95 percent of my patients wouldn't even consider trying it. The food options were not diverse, satisfying, or appealing.

Like me, my wife, Nicole, also loves good-quality food. Her father was French, and through her we have many French rela-tives who enjoy entertaining us when we visit them—and we love doing so, not just for their company but also because they invariably serve us fabulous home-cooked Mediterranean meals, reminding me of my days living on that sailboat off southern France. Inspired by these personal experi-ences, I started using my own lower-fat version of the Mediterranean diet and lifestyle instead of the Ornish plan that my patients were resisting.

My patients had been following the Standard American Diet—our mostly unhealthy Western diet commonly referred to by its all-too-appropriate acronym, SAD— loaded with processed foods, refined carbs, and unhealthy fats. As part of this new approach, they were invited to join me during group sessions with ten to twenty patients at a time. I encouraged walking and exercise, plus a diet featuring more vegetables, fruits, and beans. I allowed nuts and olive oil, but in modest proportions, and I had my patients avoid fatty dairy, fatty meats, and margarines that were popular at the time. I also gave them recipes and did cooking demonstrations for the group. This, as it turns out, was the very beginning of what would become my Mediterranean Method.

Within thirty days, my patients showed dramatic improvements in their weight, cholesterol, and blood sugar levels—in fact, many of them were able to stop their diabetic and cholesterol medications. I continued these sessions for nearly two years, and the patients continued to show amazing results and felt dramatically better. At the end, nearly half my patients who had uncontrolled diabetes, despite multiple medications, were able to stop their medications and have normal blood sugar control. The results were astonishing.

The group was asking for more recipes, and I applied for and was accepted to a chef internship at the Four Seasons restaurant in Seattle. It took me a year to complete the internship, and it really helped me learn to make food taste great. I went on to write two self-published diet-focused cookbooks.

Shortly after this experience, I became the medical director of the prestigious Pritikin Longevity Center in Miami, Florida, and I encouraged patients who had once been eating the SAD way to add more vegetables, fruits, and beans to their diet. As part of the Pritikin plan, patients were also cutting down on all fats; they showed improvements in their blood sugar and cholesterol levels, and were losing weight. Yet, this program was very similar to the ultra-low-fat Ornish program and once they left the center, almost none of my patients, nor even the staff who worked

there, could stick with this austere plan and follow it at home, on their own, over time.

Even more discouraging, in some new arrivals at the Pritikin Center who had actually already been following a Mediterranean eating plan before they got there (something we knew based on a detailed diet questionnaire they had to fill out), I noticed an increase in their blood sugar levels once they adopted this very-low-fat diet. As they cut healthy fats, such as olive oil, from their meal plan, their cholesterol profiles worsened as well, as their HDL "good" cholesterol decreased significantly.

My original goal in accepting the medical director position at Pritikin was to organize a study comparing a Mediterranean eating plan with a low-fat eating plan to measure clinical outcomes, a comparison that had yet to be made, but after a couple of years the funding for this study did not materialize. At the same time, there were new scientific studies being published that showed the real benefits of following a Mediterranean diet. Taking all this into consideration, I realized that we could do better for patients, and I created my own clinic, which became the Masley Optimal Health Center. Here I started promoting a modern-day version of the Mediterranean diet, allowing more nuts, olive oil, and avocado, as well as fatty fish; increasing the use of herbs and spices; allowing red wine and poultry in moderation; but limiting portions of carbs from rice, potatoes, and most sources of flour, including bread, pasta, and whole grains. The Mediterranean Method was coming into sharper focus.

Why did I tweak the traditional Mediterranean diet for my patients, cutting back on the breads and pastas we tend to think of as Mediterranean? Because for the most part, my patients were not active for six to ten hours per day, harvesting crops or fishing the sea like traditional Mediterranean basin laborers. They worked in offices and had indoor jobs where they sat for most of the day, and they were struggling to get four to seven hours of activity per week, not per day. Their bodies weren't able to handle excess portions of carbohydrates (even from "healthy" whole grains). I wanted to take their modern lifestyles into account, and so I updated an ancient diet for modern times.

Not only did their food—with all its wonderful Mediterranean flavors—taste far better than what they had been eating but also at my clinic we achieved even better results than I had hoped. Over the last fifteen years, I've published results showing that my average patient had lost weight, had improved blood sugar, blood pressure, and cholesterol levels, and more important, had also reduced their arterial plaque load and improved their brain processing speed. (I'll expand on how we measured this and the results in later chapters.) My average patient was physiologically ten years younger after adopting my Mediterranean recommendations.

My goal in *The Mediterranean Method* is to help you bring the healthiest version of a Mediterranean diet into your own kitchen and adopt a way of eating—along with a stress-free, joy-filled attitude toward food and cooking—that will benefit you and anyone else who sits at your table. Beyond its healthy appeal, there is another reason I'm such an advocate for the Mediterranean diet: The food tastes fantastic, which is why this diet is perhaps the easiest of all to follow, and to stick with—for life.

What You'll Find in *The Mediterranean Method*

NOW THAT YOU know why I'm so enthusiastic about this way of eating, I'll tell you more about its origins and basic principles in the chapters that follow—including more specific guidelines on what constitutes an authentic Mediterranean diet (and what foods do not), as well as which nutrients in these foods are likely responsible for the longevity and excellent health of people who eat and live the Mediterranean way. You also learn about the active but relaxed lifestyle that complements this diet.

We'll look at how these foods specifically boost weight loss, cardiovascular health, cognitive function, and your gut microbiome, as well as reduce the risk of chronic disease and extend your life span. And at the heart of it all is my Mediterranean Method—a "skinny twist" on Mediterranean eating. With the information in this book, you can make the Mediterranean diet yours—and get healthier with every breakfast, lunch, and dinner you eat, as well as snacks.

I'll help you clean out your cabinets and restock them with staples that you'll want to cook with and eat, and I'll give you tips on what kinds of fresh foods you should have on hand. You may not be able to shop for provisions in a French market, but these days you can do pretty well at your local grocery store, once you know what to put in your cart! Finally, I'll give you 50 easy-to-use, flavorful recipes that you can enjoy and share with friends and family. Best of all, *you can start eating this way today.* Just keep reading.

I won't ever forget what a wise mentor once told me when I was a premed student trying to plan my classes and map out my future in medicine. This was well before I had immersed myself in studies on nutrition and health, before I'd researched and seen firsthand how it is possible to prevent and/or reverse so much of the chronic disease that plagues us—and how food is central to our well-being.

"If you want to make a difference as a doctor and truly benefit the health of your patients," my college adviser told me, "write a cookbook. Instead of writing them prescriptions for medications—give them recipes!" This book offers you 50 recipes—but it's much more than a cookbook. Consider it a prescription for a lifestyle that's not only delicious and easy to follow but also healthy, with

lifelong benefits for mind and body. It's the fruit of my labors both as a doctor and as a trained chef.

As I write this, I'm preparing to set off on another journey with my wife aboard our sailboat, once again exploring the coastal regions of the Mediterranean Sea and all that it offers—not just the gorgeous vistas and welcoming people but also the wonderful bounty of beautiful, fresh foods that make up the Mediterranean diet at its very best. If I can prepare these meals in a small sailboat galley, then certainly you should be able to make them in your home. I wish you happy and healthy eating!

MY PROMISE TO YOU

In *The Mediterranean Method*, I'll offer you:

- A delicious variety of foods that you and your family will love.

- A medically sound plan that will help you be trim and slim.

- A scientifically proven program that will dramatically reduce your risk for heart attacks and strokes, memory loss, and cancer.

- Tips that will also make you fitter, in mind and body, with less stress.

- 50 recipes to get you on your way that are fun to prepare.

- A plan that will extend your longevity, *joie de vivre*, and help you to feel better than you have in over a decade.

1

A WHOLE-FOODS DIET FOR THE WHOLE PLANET

When you think of the "Mediterranean diet," what comes to mind? In my experience, people seem to dwell on a handful of notions. *It's olive oil and red wine . . . lots of garlic and tomatoes . . . seafood . . . pasta? . . . It's vaguely Italian, French, Greek, or Spanish. . . .* None of those ideas are wrong, nor are they completely accurate—because they don't tell the whole story of this ancient way of eating, nor do they reveal the full, flavorful bounty of this diet, one that is as healthy as it is delicious. For thousands of years, people along the Mediterranean coastline have shared many of the same dietary staples—especially olives and olive oil, fish and seafood, a lush bounty of fresh vegetables in every color of the rainbow, juicy ripe fruits (including grapes for eating and wine-making), nuts, beans, legumes, and whole grains.

We tend to think of Western European countries—most notably France, Italy, Spain, and Greece—as the originators of the Mediterranean diet, but given the centuries-old, cross-cultural history of the region, as well as a shared climate and similar growing seasons, you'll find some of the same foods served in North African and Middle Eastern countries as well. Portugal's coastline is primarily Atlantic, but there they follow many classic variations on the Mediterranean diet.

And from region to region, these variations only broaden the possibilities of the flavors you'll encounter—French thyme instead of rosemary, garlic-roasted eggplant served with couscous instead of grilled zucchini and pasta, Greek feta instead of Spanish manchego, and so on. The breadth of fresh, simple flavors and their mouth-watering possibilities make this diet versatile and appealing, and it has long been associated with excellent health and longevity.

What's the other reason why the nutrient-rich traditional Mediterranean diet is synonymous with wellness? It's because of what people *don't* eat. Red meat is uncommon, and processed meats even rarer. Processed foods, including refined carbohydrates loaded with artificial flavorings, are almost nonexistent. Sugary treats are reserved for celebrations. Serving sizes, including protein portions, are smaller than what we are used to.

On top of that, Mediterranean people are physically active, every single day, and have a strong sense of community and connection. They enjoy life, they enjoy real food, and they enjoy sharing it with others. Combine a delicious diet and a less stressful, happier way of living, and the result is this: people who are trim and fit, with lower rates of chronic disease and longer life spans.

But here's the thing: You don't have to live in the Mediterranean to enjoy the health-boosting benefits of this delicious food and leisurely lifestyle. You can eat and live this way wherever you call home. *The Mediterranean Method* is designed to help you embrace this traditional diet in a practical, modern way—to help you get healthy, and stay that way. Whether or not you've ventured abroad, you deserve to know more about the true Mediterranean diet and its benefits, a way of eating—and living—that is linked to record levels of longevity and low rates of chronic disease. And in contrast to all the crazy fad diets that have come and gone over the last couple of decades, this one has been around for thousands of years.

Diving into the Mediterranean— and the Blue Zones Beyond

THERE ARE MORE than a few misconceptions about the Mediterranean diet—and the lifestyle that goes with it—starting with the name itself. While the Mediterranean Basin is indeed where you'll find most of the people who enjoy this food, as discussed earlier, it's not strictly European. You'll find followers of a Mediterranean diet in Portugal, North African countries such as Morocco and Tunisia, and Middle Eastern regions, including Turkey, Egypt, Israel, Lebanon, and Syria.

Farther afield, you'll find a very similar style of eating and living—lots of plant foods, healthy fats, little (if any) red meat, plenty of physical activity—in communities as diverse as Loma Linda, California; Okinawa,

Japan; and the Nicoya Peninsula of Costa Rica. What do those far-flung locales have in common with Mediterranean regions? Like places such as the Italian island of Sardinia and the Greek island of Ikaria, they are all considered "Blue Zones," the name given to at least five specific regions around the world by a team of researchers, led by *National Geographic* writer Dan Buettner, who have set out to chronicle the habits of the healthiest and longest-lived people around the globe.

The Blue Zones are home to communities of individuals who routinely live without disease well into their 80s, 90s, and beyond. Interestingly, while there are marked variations in what Blue Zone dwellers eat based on their location, there are more similarities than differences.

Loma Linda is home to a large community of Seventh-day Adventists, many of whom are descendants of the original founders of the church itself. For religious reasons, they are vegetarian and eat far more plants than animal foods, which are limited to eggs and dairy. The residents of Okinawa are famous for their robust health and low rates of heart disease, cancer, and dementia—the women there live longer than women anywhere else on earth—and they eat lots of vegetables and fish. The people of Nicoya, Costa Rica, are active outdoors like their Mediterranean counterparts—getting much needed vitamin D from the sun—and they build their diets around a traditional dish of fiber-rich beans, vegetables, and whole grains, as well as some dairy.

Of course, there are significant differences. Unlike people along the Mediterranean, Loma Linda residents eat very little seafood, Okinawans consume lots

of fermented foods such as soy products, and the whole grain of choice in Costa Rica is corn. But despite such variations, there are overlapping themes with the plant-rich Mediterranean diet, with foods such as green leafy vegetables, nuts, beans, and fish.

Travel back to the Mediterranean region and you'll find the famed Blue Zone of Sardinia, home to a relatively high proportion of centenarians who are the source of much curiosity. What's their secret? Besides their active lifestyle and connection to community and family, Sardinians are famous for their production (and consumption) of a particular type of native red wine, Cannonau, that is high in polyphenols, the antioxidant compounds that give red wine its proven protective benefits, especially with regard to heart disease. But it isn't just this special red wine that make them live so long and healthy, as Sardinians also follow a traditional Mediterranean diet very closely, which likely provides the greatest benefit.

The other well-known Mediterranean Blue Zone is the Greek island of Ikaria, dubbed "the island where people forgot to die." Interestingly, one researcher points out that their consumption of polyphenols—not from wine but from a diverse array of herbs like wild mint and rosemary—probably plays a role in their good health and lack of disease.

It seems that wherever they live, however they compose their meals based on geography or ethnicity, availability of foods, and tradition, followers of a Mediterranean-style diet have much in common when they choose what to eat: plentiful fiber-packed vegetables and fruits, nuts, flavors from healthy fats, herbs and spices, little to no red meat, clean protein such as fresh seafood, beans and legumes, some dairy, moderate amounts of organically raised poultry and eggs, and whole grains. And we can zero in on the Mediterranean region specifically for extra-virgin olive oil as a healthy fat, along with moderate consumption of red wine.

While the diets of people in non-Mediterranean Blue Zones are clearly beneficial, based on my experience—as a physician advocating for health through nutrition, and as a trained chef who loves to make delicious meals—I always return to the original Mediterranean diet, with its straight-forward emphasis on seasonal whole foods. The reason why I recommend it to patients and serve it at my table to friends and family is simple: It's the easiest, healthiest, and best-tasting diet to follow on the planet.

More Than an Ancient Diet for Modern Times

I WASN'T ALWAYS a champion of the Mediterranean diet. In fact, as I mentioned earlier, I was the medical director for the Pritikin Longevity Center years ago, and I reluctantly advocated an ultra-low-fat eating plan with very little protein and almost no fat. The Pritikin plan, like the Mediterranean diet, featured lots of vegetables, whole high-fiber foods, and no processed or refined carbohydrates. But the similarities ended there. One major difference? The Pritikin plan was extremely hard to follow. With hardly any fat, it lacked flavor and a pleasant mouthfeel that comes with eating fat; and with very limited protein, it didn't satisfy hunger adequately. For those reasons, it failed to have the lasting benefits I'd hoped for.

Years later, I designed a diet for patients at my clinic, the Masley Optimal Health Center, that included a Mediterranean eating plan with lots of fiber, clean protein (including fish and seafood), and good amounts of healthy fat, as well as ample herbs and spices. This would become the basis of my Mediterranean Method. The diet was simple to follow, the foods tasted wonderful, and the results were excellent. Patients lost weight and improved their cholesterol levels, and they felt better overall. I also was reminded of how much this diet echoed the food I'd shopped for, cooked, and enjoyed when I'd lived and worked in the South of France as a student.

After observing the health benefits of the Mediterranean diet firsthand for over thirty-plus years, and seeing patients prevent and reverse heart disease, inflammation, metabolic syndrome, and cognitive dysfunc-tion, I know it's not merely an ancient diet for modern times; when properly applied, it's also an ancient antidote for modern disease.

What to Eat, Starting Now

IT'S EASY TO describe the Mediterranean diet, but despite its simplicity, it's also important to "translate" or adapt it for Americans because we live such different lifestyles, starting with our physical activity—or rather, alas, our inactivity. Even if we work out, we aren't nearly as active as people in the Mediterranean. Consider a farmer who is physically active eight hours a day, or even a city dweller who cycles or walks to her job. On average, Americans struggle to get seven-plus hours of physical activity per *week*. We don't walk to work or work the land. We mostly buy our food in grocery stores, not outdoor markets or specialty shops. And the food itself may not be as fresh or nutrient-packed as what someone can harvest from a farmer's organic garden down the road, or purchase from the local fish market within view of the sea. But it's still very possible to re-create this diet and bring the Mediterranean home, starting with how you compose your very next meal.

You've probably seen popular Mediterranean diet pyramids that echo what we've been discussing: an emphasis on lots of fruits and vegetables, healthy fats from olive oil and nuts, whole grains, fish and seafood, some dairy and poultry, and very little red meat or sweets, as well as red wine.

Plant-based foods are always the foundation and therefore are the largest building block of this food pyramid, with animal products—including dairy—given less emphasis as you move to the top. This is a reflection of how people who traditionally consumed the Mediterranean diet sourced their food—straight from the land or pulled from the sea. You may have enough good food in your kitchen right now to make your next meal a Mediterranean-style one. Always start with plant foods and build your plate on that foundation. Here's my Mediterranean Method version:

A FEW TIMES PER MONTH
red meat, sweets, flour products, potatoes

SEVERAL TIMES (3–5) PER WEEK
fish and seafood, poultry, eggs, whole grains, probiotic-rich dairy (including cheese)

DAILY
vegetables, fruits, beans, nuts, olive oil and other smart fats, herbs and spices, yogurt, dark chocolate, red wine, coffee, tea, water

FOUNDATION
outdoor activity and exercise, market shopping, group cooking, relaxation, leisurely dining with social interaction, and mindful eating

Most space is taken up by your daily essentials, and the middle represents foods you should have three to five times per week. There are few "forbidden foods" on the Mediterranean diet (except for the obvious, such as chemical artificial flavorings, animal protein injected with hormones, or toxic trans fats), but the top of the pyramid represents foods most people should have a few times a month, as opposed to every day or several times during the week.

And note the bottom layer that supports this whole approach: a less stressful lifestyle of activity and social connection.

In the next chapter, we'll look closer at each component of a Mediterranean-style diet and you'll get answers to the questions you'll undoubtedly want answered, on topics ranging from serving sizes to substitutions; from how often to eat certain foods in the weekly category to whether or not you can

eat unlimited quantities from the daily; from whether or not to buy organic to what kind of tea or dark chocolate. *What*, you may be wondering, *is a Mediterranean breakfast? And can I still have my protein shake in the morning? Why aren't whole grains eaten every day? What is a serving size? Should I aim for certain amounts of proteins, fats, and carbohydrates? How much wine can I have? I don't drink alcohol (or coffee)—what should I do? What are other examples of smart fats besides olive oil? How do I modify this plan if I want to lose weight? If I'm more active, can I have more whole grains per week?* (Short answer to that one: yes.)

Rest assured, your questions will be answered, you'll know what and how much to eat, and your kitchen will eventually be so well stocked that you're never at a loss for meal ideas. Best of all, you'll be highly satisfied—and healthier.

Before You Begin (what *not* to do)

IF YOU WANT to "go Mediterranean" with your very next meal, by now you should have some general ideas—and inspiration—on where to start. Before we move on to the nitty-gritty on how to choose the right mix of foods for your needs and how to sustain this diet for the long term, let's take a closer look at some common errors many people make

when they try this approach. Suppose you're heading into the kitchen or sitting down at your table with the best of intentions, but the results of doing one or more of the following can be an unhealthy undoing of the Mediterranean diet.

MISTAKE #1. IGNORING PORTION CONTROL (YOU CAN EAT TOO MUCH "HEALTHY" FOOD!)

Even when we're talking about smart fats, such as olive oil and nuts, portion control is always important, especially if you're trying to lose weight. There's no need to put a hard limit on daily servings of vegetables (you won't overdo it because you'll naturally fill up on fiber), but it is possible, for instance, to overeat walnuts or almond butter, or use too much olive oil, particularly if you're dipping pieces of bread into it. (Speaking of bread, see below.) Be mindful. (And for the record, one serving of nuts is about 1 to 2 handfuls, the amount you can hold in the palm of your hand, and a serving of olive oil is typically 1 to 2 tablespoons per person per dish.)

MISTAKE #2. OVERDOING GRAINS AND CEREALS (INCLUDING BREAD AND PASTA)

Because most of us aren't as active as our Mediterranean counterparts, we can't justify serving ourselves enormous portions of grains and cereals. Unlike them, we haven't "earned" larger servings. The Mediterranean diet has been eaten traditionally by people who were physically active most of their waking hours—not just fishermen and farmers but also city dwellers who walk everywhere. We get into our cars and drive a few blocks to the supermarket, but Europeans walk to work (or to the metro), to school, to the shops and markets, and through parks, plazas, and piazzas. In Italy, the *passegiata*—an evening stroll before or after dinner—is a must, and in

every country you'll find that daily walking is fundamental. Here we have to count our steps with a pedometer or an app to make sure we're getting enough activity!

When you see grains and cereals on the Mediterranean diet, this doesn't mean a giant platter of pasta, unlimited bread (even if it's organic and whole grain), or bowls of rice (even if it's brown rice). It's important to control your portions of grains and cereals—for reasons I'll detail in Chapter 2—and as you'll see, of all the foods listed in the Mediterranean diet, whole grains provide the least benefit. (And incidentally, even those farmers and fishermen aren't eating super-sized American portions of pasta, polenta, and rice.)

MISTAKE #3. NOT EATING ENOUGH FISH AND SEAFOOD

Eating fish merely a few times a month won't yield the disease-fighting benefits of the Mediterranean diet, particularly for the heart and brain. Aim for seafood at least twice a week—preferably three to five times per week. If you're concerned about how to shop for and prepare fish (or if you think it's too expensive or you're concerned about mercury), you'll find answers to all your questions, including recipes, in later chapters. And if you are vegetarian, or you've declared yourself to be a person who "hates" seafood, in the name of your health and longevity, it is possible to supplement with fish oil (see page 87) or seaweed oil. However, in most studies, the long-chain omega-3 fats you get from consuming fish and shellfish—as well as foods such as seaweed—are more beneficial to your brain and body than such supplements alone.

MISTAKE #4. THINKING THAT ALL CHEESES (AND YOGURTS) ARE CREATED EQUAL

Dairy isn't heavily emphasized on the Mediterranean diet, but it is a healthy part of it. However, treating pasteurized cheese as a go-to food—compared, for example, with raw, probiotic-rich and vitamin K_2-loaded camembert—is a mistake. A cellophane-wrapped, mass-produced cheese stick might have to do if you're stuck without any other food and your blood sugar is on a roller-coaster ride, but it's not as nutrient-rich (or as deliciously satisfying) as a small serving of the camembert—or a bit of fresh mozzarella, aged manchego, or tangy feta. The same goes for yogurt. Sugary, artificially flavored yogurt hardly has anything in common—or any benefits, especially for your gut health—compared to plain Greek-style yogurt or kefir that you can flavor yourself with fresh fruit, some walnuts, and optionally, a bit of honey. Many of my patients are shocked when I explain that fruit-flavored yogurt has more sugar than ice cream. As with so many components of the Mediterranean diet, when choosing your foods, simple is best.

MISTAKE #5. SKIPPING THE BEANS

As with fish, many folks forgo the beans: *They take too long to make . . . They give me gas . . . I don't know which ones to buy . . . I don't like them . . . Paleo diets forbid them. . . .* Don't miss out on this fiber-packed super-food that, as you'll learn later, is one of the best foods for controlling blood sugar, and it's the #1 all-time top food for blocking

disease-causing oxidation. In Mediterranean cuisine, beans can become the healthy foundation for countless meals. You'll find recipes to incorporate them into your diet in Chapter 9, such as my Spanish White Bean Soup (page 178) or my side dish of fava beans and chard with roasted tomato, onion, and garlic (see page 218), but you can enjoy some Mediterranean flavors at your next lunch or dinner without a lot of effort.

Try this simple idea now: Combine mixed greens with canned garbanzo beans, halved cherry tomatoes, some slivers of red onion, and a handful of fresh herbs. Squeeze some fresh lemon on top, drizzle with extra-virgin olive oil, toss to combine, and season to taste with sea salt and freshly ground pepper. You can add some sliced chicken, a hard-boiled egg, or some fish for added protein. For a Greek twist, use some olives and a touch of crumbled feta.

MISTAKE #6. TAKING SHORTCUTS WITH PROCESSED FOODS

Canned beans are but one example of a healthy shortcut you can take on your way to a Mediterranean diet, especially if you're pressed for time. (Choose BPA-free cans; see note on page 26.) But a fast-food fried fish sandwich is not, nor is a pepperoni pizza, or that box of garlic-flavored instant couscous. Refined carbohydrates, unhealthy fats such as trans fats, and risky preservatives, artificial sweeteners, and other chemical additives that can damage your health are impossible to avoid if you eat processed foods—and some people do so because they're rushed at meal-time. But buying the additive-packed "instant" version or choosing fast food as a shortcut is a bad bet in the long run. Chemically loaded processed foods are not a part of a Mediterranean diet or my version of it. (And canned beans are not a processed food—but they are a healthy option that will save you hours of cooking time.)

Why You Should Choose BPA-free Cans

The Mediterranean eating style features foods such as beans and tomato products that are conveniently available on your supermarket shelves—but choose BPA-free canned food containers, or buy these foods in glass jars. Bisphenol A (BPA) is an environmental toxin that has been shown to increase the risk for chronic disease, including high blood pressure, diabetes, and cancer. Just two servings per week of food from cans and containers containing BPA can cause this chemical to build up in your system and cause harm. It is used in the manufacturing of plastics, including plastic food wrap and storage containers—and it was actually used in baby bottles until consumers pushed back. BPA is an "endocrine disruptor," meaning that it can interfere with normal hormonal activity in your body. (It actually mimics the activity of estrogen, and has been associated with early puberty in girls.) Even though it's still widely used in consumer products, don't let this powerful chemical into your food supply—and your body.

MISTAKE #7. DRINKING TOO MUCH WINE (AND NOT ENOUGH WATER)

Alcohol is not a staple of the Mediterranean eating style, though much has been made of its benefits. However, understand that *the only alcohol with proven health benefits is red wine.* Not beer, not gin, nor tequila. And white wine has fewer benefits than red wine. Yet, red wine only provides health benefits if it is consumed in moderation. Enjoy a glass or two with dinner, but quench your thirst with water. In Mediterranean Europe, diners go through more bottles of mineral water than they do wine—and not just in the hot summer months. But filtered tap water works just as well! (You'll learn more about the beneficial compounds in red wine in the chapters to come.)

MISTAKE #8. HIGH-HEAT COOKING WITH EXTRA-VIRGIN OLIVE OIL

Don't use extra-virgin olive oil for high-heat cooking, or even medium-high heat. Once it reaches 400°F—its smoke point, the maximum temperature it can reach before it breaks down and becomes a damaged fat—extra-virgin olive oil starts losing nutritional value, not to mention its complex and delicate flavors. Even worse, heat-damaged oils oxidize and become pro-inflammatory. Overheating good olive oil is not just a health risk; it's also a waste of money. Save flavorful extra-virgin olive oil for drizzling over foods and making dressings, and use virgin olive oil and a handful of others (such as avocado and/or almond oil) for medium-high cooking. (For more details see page 34.)

MISTAKE #9. LIMITING YOUR PALATE

One reason it's easy to adapt the Mediterranean diet to our American palate is that we're already enjoying some of these flavors. We are, after all, a nation of immigrants (many of whom came from not only southern Italy, Spain, France, and Greece but also Turkey, the Middle East, and Northern Africa), and as a nation we celebrate many traditional cuisines. Garlic—one of the hallmark flavors of this food and a powerful anti-inflammatory—is hardly an exotic ingredient! Still, don't limit yourself to the "safe" and familiar flavors of Mediterranean cuisine from Western Europe. Remember the influences from North Africa, Turkey, Israel, and other Middle Eastern regions, where you'll

find spices such as inflammation-fighting turmeric and gut-healthy fermented foods like kefir (which originated in Russia). Tomatoes, chili peppers, sweet potatoes, avocados, dark chocolate, and many other beneficial foods originally hail from Southeast Asia, Africa, Latin America, and parts of the globe that are far from the Mediterranean.

The recipes beginning on page 163 emphasize Mediterranean foods, but don't be surprised if you see an infusion of flavors that you wouldn't expect to find in that region. If you remain open to new flavors and ingredients with proven health benefits, you're not only broadening your palate and enjoying new foods, you're increasing your chances of preventing chronic disease and living a longer, happier life.

Some Important Do's—and One Final Don't

ABOVE ALL, *do enjoy your food*. Do take pleasure in rediscovering the fun of gathering wonderful ingredients to prepare a simple meal, one that will benefit you—mind, body, and soul.

But don't ignore what happens away from the table, outside the kitchen. As mentioned earlier, the Mediterranean diet isn't just about food. It's a whole lifestyle. Being physically active every day, reducing stress and feeling rested, having social connections, and

adopting a more joyful and relaxed attitude about eating are as important as what is on your plate. These themes will come up again and again as you learn more about the wonders of the Mediterranean diet, but you'll only reap its full benefits if you embrace all its facets—beyond food. Fortunately, any lifestyle modifications you make will be as enjoyable as the food is delicious.

2

HOW TO EAT: A NEW MEDITERRANEAN DIET

The all-American plate has looked the same for generations. It's a meal built around a generous quantity of a specific animal protein: beef, chicken, pork, or fish, accompanied by a large starchy side such as rice, noodles, or mashed potatoes and a modest serving of green vegetables, almost as a garnish. And often there is dessert.

Most Americans grew up eating some version of that classic meat-and-potatoes dinner, and they have continued to do so into adulthood, whether they cook at home or eat out. We've updated the protein, exchanging Mom's humble pot roast for trendy flatiron steak, or Dad's favorite pork chop for pork tenderloin. The side dish is more sophisticated, too—orzo or couscous, or oven-roasted potatoes. The vegetables aren't the infamous canned varieties we had to choke down in order to earn dessert, but the serving size of plant foods remains meager. (And don't forget dessert.)

The irony is that today's family dinner may be less bland than the "square meal" once considered healthy and wholesome—but the too-large portions and ratios of animal protein to plants, with lots of starchy carbs, are not an improvement. Even worse, much more of our food is processed with loads of harmful additives that cancel out nutritional value. If we're cooking at home, at least we have some control—but sometimes we're "cooking" frozen entrees made with an endless list of ingredients, with instant, artificially flavored side dishes straight out of a box. And frequently, we're relying on fast-food or restaurant meals. It doesn't matter that we've updated our foods and flavors for the twenty-first century. We're *still* eating last century's Standard American Diet (SAD)—and it's making us fat and sick.

Even less healthy is the snacking that happens between meals (and even after dinner and dessert). For the average American, snacking adds an extra 600 to 900 calories to our waistline every day. Instead of eating mindfully, oftentimes snacking occurs in front of the television, or while standing in front of the refrigerator or cupboard in the kitchen with some of the worst options: candy, sodas, cookies, peanuts, ice cream, mints, chips, and crackers.

Contrast our SAD approach with the Mediterranean diet, where a dinner plate—or even a series of small plates—looks very different from the SAD protein/starch/vegetable template. And it tastes different, too—it tastes *better*. As you know by now, a typical Mediterranean meal is plant-based, with generous portion sizes for salads, vegetable dishes, beans, and perhaps a smaller portion of a whole grain. Fifty to 65 percent of the time—not at every meal—there will be a 4- to 5-ounce portion of animal protein. Because of the built-in variety the food is colorful and its fresh flavors are diverse and satisfying. And often there is dessert—but it is typically a serving of fruit or dark chocolate, occasionally a dessert flavored with honey.

As for snacking? It's not an ingrained habit as it is in this country, and in fact for the most part, it's frowned upon. Eating is done at a table, with others, and as a result, Europeans snack far less.

The bottom line is that you eat less with the Mediterranean Method than you do on a SAD diet—and yet the food is so fantastic that you are more satisfied.

This chapter is your guide to foods you'll find on a traditional Mediterranean diet, and it will give you a basis for how to put all your meals together, with or without a recipe. You'll also notice that I've "edited" this traditional approach for the twenty-first century, compared to what you might see on a typical Mediterranean diet pyramid—changes I've made to help us overcome the damage done by generations of SAD eating. Is it possible to improve upon the world's healthiest diet? Depending on your health goals and how you choose to use the Mediterranean Method, the answer may be . . . yes.

The Food: Everyday Essentials

**Vegetables, fruits, beans, nuts,
olive oil and other smart fats,
herbs and spices, yogurt and/or kefir,
dark chocolate, red wine, coffee, tea**
Consider these foods a foundation—and the makings of your grocery list—and aim to eat them every day. A note on recommended servings: You don't have to strictly limit the amounts of plant foods such as vegetables and beans, especially when they're the basis of a meal. It's hard to overeat vegetables, for instance, so you'll naturally limit yourself. What's a bigger issue, I have found, is getting people to eat the *minimum* amounts of plant foods recommended here. My recipes will help you reach your goal of incorporating these foods into your daily diet, and will inspire you to try your own flavor combinations.

VEGETABLES AND FRUITS:
**5 cups/day
(1 medium piece of fruit = 1 cup)**

The Basics
If you're picturing your plate, most of it should be plant-based foods, including vegetables and fruits. Aim for more vegetables than fruit, since they have almost no impact on blood sugar levels. Keep in mind that a ripe banana or potatoes can send your blood sugar soaring, especially first thing in the morning when we are more sensitive to carbs,

while a half cup of berries or a serving of broccoli any time of day won't increase your blood sugar levels in any noticeable way. As you will discover soon, some forms of produce have a bigger impact on blood sugar levels than others. At lunch and dinner, enjoy the range of nutrient-packed plant pigments and fiber you'll find in a range of vegetables—not just the greens and leafy greens but also the oranges, reds, and yellows.

The Extras
As mentioned, ripe bananas can have a big impact on blood sugar, and that's also true for dried fruits and fruit juice, which have high concentrations of fructose. Treat them as occasional foods, and exchange fruit juice for a piece of whole fruit. Fiber-packed berries and cherries are especially good choices because they're packed with beneficial anti-inflammatory and anti-oxidant flavonoids. Stir them into probiotic-rich yogurt or enjoy them with some dark chocolate for dessert.

Just a reminder that when it comes to vegetables, enjoy a wide variety and don't be concerned about limiting yourself—it's getting to a minimum that's a bigger challenge. The only vegetable to treat as an occasional food is the starchy potato, which has a high sugar-load and will impact your blood sugar levels accordingly. (See page 52 for ways to reduce potatoes' impact on blood sugar.)

There are few fruits and vegetables that won't grow in temperate Mediterranean climates, though some are distinctly more native than others or are closely associated with the cuisine of the region—tomatoes, leafy greens, onions, zucchini, citrus, and of course, grapes and olives are high on the long list! If you walk through a market in France, Spain, Italy, or Greece, depending on the season, you'll find an astounding range of produce, because it truly is the foundation for Mediterranean meals. If I had to narrow down my favorite fruit and vegetable choices for smart nutrition delivered with maximum flavor, it would be: berries, cherries, apples, pears, oranges, and figs (fresh, not dried); kale, arugula (called "rocket" in Europe), spinach, broccoli, fennel, tomatoes, onion, artichokes, and asparagus.

BEANS:
1 serving (½ cup/day)

The Basics
The humble bean packs a powerful nutritional punch, boasting plenty of potassium, magnesium, mixed folates, and B vitamins. Beans, which are also a lean protein source, are a mainstay of almost all Mediterranean cuisines. Some classic examples are chickpeas (garbanzo beans), white beans (cannellini), fava beans, green beans (haricots verts), and lentils (French green or any variety)—but of course there are also kidney, pinto, butter, and black beans, plus dozens of other varieties to choose from, including Japanese edamame (soy)beans, which offer the most protein. Garbanzos can be used whole on salads or puréed, to make hummus (see recipe, page 229). You can enjoy beans on their own as a side dish (try my Roasted Garbanzo

Beans as an appetizer, page 171), or use them as a basis for a main dish. See the White Bean and Celery Salad (page 186).

The Extras
You can make home-cooked beans—it's easier than you think. I've included simple instructions on preparing dried beans—see the recipe for Spanish White Bean Soup (page 178). You can cook beans on your stovetop, in a pressure cooker, or in a slow cooker—or simply use canned. Choose BPA-free cans, or look for varieties sold in glass. Cooked beans freeze well, so it's easy to keep a supply on hand for daily consumption.

NUTS:
1–2 servings (1–2 handfuls/day)

The Basics
Nuts—as well as seeds—are a healthy fat. (See page 159—nuts can count toward your daily 4 to 6 servings of healthy fats.) Almonds, walnuts, pistachios, filberts, macadamias, and pecans are all terrific choices, as they provide healthy fats (that play a beneficial role in heart and brain health), as well as fiber, folate, vitamin E, and a bit of protein. Nuts can be eaten as a snack, but they are commonly served as a garnish for many dishes, including salads, grain dishes, breakfast (see Berries and Yogurt with Toasted Muesli, page 165), and even a coating over fish and poultry.

The Extras
A "handful" is exactly that—it's the amount of nuts that you can cup in the palm of your hand. If you're petite, it's a smaller handful than for someone who is larger. Nuts have

many benefits and can help in improving cholesterol profiles, balancing blood sugar and curbing hunger (eating a couple handfuls once or twice per day is associated with losing weight), but they aren't a low-calorie food, so if you're trying to lose weight, be mindful about what one to two "handfuls" is for you; it doesn't mean eat the whole 16-ounce can.

Peanuts are a legume (as are beans), not a nut. They aren't unhealthy, but they don't fall into the same category as nuts in terms of their benefits.

Besides eating whole nuts, try nut butters. Almond butter on apple slices or with celery sticks is a satisfying afternoon snack with contrast and crunch. If you want to make your own almond butter at home, process roasted almonds in a food processor until smooth and add a bit of salt to taste. (Try toasting raw almonds or already-roasted almonds and process when they're still warm for faster results.) Tahini, not a nut butter but made from sesame seeds, is another good choice and brings a bit of the Middle Eastern influence into your Mediterranean diet. (See the Method Hummus on page 229 as an example.)

OLIVE OILS AND OTHER SMART FATS: 4-6 servings per day

The Basics

If there is one iconic ingredient of the Mediterranean diet, it's olive oil. Olive oil is strongly associated with the well-documented heart-healthy paybacks of the Mediterranean diet, but there is significant research on its other benefits as well, including its brain-boosting benefits and its role in preserving cognitive function as we age. You'll learn more about the cardiovascular benefits of olive oil in Chapter 4.

There are two mistakes many Americans make with olive oil when they're incorporating it into their daily diets. The first is cooking with it at high heat (see later and page 26). The second is using too little or too much of it. One serving of olive oil is typically 1 to 2 tablespoons per person per dish. That may not sound like much, but if you're consuming it "straight" (not cooking with it), then a tablespoon or two per person will go a long way toward flavoring fresh foods, and published studies show that consuming up to ½ cup of olive oil per person per day is associated with weight loss and better health. Still, it's not hard to pour ½ cup of oil into a single recipe if you're not paying attention. (A tablespoon of any oil has 120 calories, which is reasonable, while ½ cup provides 960 calories, which 2–3 times per day would be over the top.) And take note of how some foods absorb it more rapidly than others (such as eggplant). It's still there even if you don't see it! Just 1 to 2 tablespoons in a serving of food can provide a wonderful smooth texture and a lovely flavor.

Olive oil, of course, isn't the only smart-healthy fat. Besides nuts (see earlier), seeds also are an excellent source of healthy fats and nutrients. Pumpkin seeds, for instance, are rich in magnesium—a nutrient necessary for heart health that many of us are deficient in. Sunflower seeds are loaded with vitamin E. Flax and chia seeds—though not traditional Mediterranean diet foods—are also good picks. One serving of seeds is 1 tablespoon, or 1 ounce per person.

Potassium-packed avocados, high in fiber

and heart-healthy fats, can also be part of a Mediterranean diet, and because of their popularity in this country, they're easy to find in your local market year-round. Combine cubed avocado with sliced cherry tomatoes, some chickpeas, a drizzle of olive oil, sea salt, pepper, and some lemon or lime juice—simple and satisfying. (One half of an avocado is one serving of smart fat.)

The Extras
(especially the extra-virgin extras)

Do not use olive oil for high-heat cooking. As discussed in Chapter 1, high heat obliterates its nutrients and even turns it into an unhealthy fat. It also destroys the taste—making it bitter, another reason why it's a waste of money to ruin your good oil with high heat. Reserve *extra-virgin olive oil* for low-heat cooking, as well as salads or dressings; and use *virgin olive oil* for medium-high cooking (since virgin olive oil may be difficult to find, for high-heat cooking, you can also use avocado oil, almond oil, or ghee). Avoid regular *processed olive oil*, as chemicals and heat are used to extract the oil; the result is damaged oil that is contaminated with chemical residues. (For information on other healthy fats for cooking, including the smoke points for olive oil and other cooking oils and fats, see page 26.)

Beware of suspiciously cheap olive oil. It's likely adulterated with other oils such as soybean or canola oils, or it may not actually be extra-virgin. Extra-virgin is made through the first pressing of the olives without heat or chemicals; virgin olive oil (which can be used for medium-high cooking) is generally not obtained from the first pressing, or depending on the grower/bottler, it could be made from olives that aren't considered as high-grade and superior as those used to make extra-virgin oil. Regular processed olive oil, sometimes labeled as "pure" or "light" (but never "virgin"), is closely related to other refined, unhealthy cooking oils in that it's produced with heat that damages the oil, and perhaps with chemical additives.

Much has been made of the origins of olive oil and where the "best" oil comes from. It's largely a matter of taste—and also availability. Italian olive oil has long been prized for its quality, but weather extremes in recent years have damaged harvests and dramatically impacted that country's yields. Spain, Portugal, Greece, California, and most recently Tunisia also produce significant volumes of high-quality extra-virgin olive oil. In fact, Spain—home to the healthiest, longest-lived people in the Western world—is the largest producer of olive oil and offers one of my personal favorites. France, Turkey, and even Australia also produce high-quality olive oils.

Some bottlers sell a "blend" of extra-virgin olive oils from different countries, but buyer beware: If it's sold in a giant plastic jug container, and it's really cheap, it's probably not the real McCoy. (Some reports suggest that up to half of all olive oil from Europe has been diluted with cheaper, less healthy oils.) Ideally, look for some form of certification, such as the California Olive Oil Council, to ensure that you are getting the real thing.

In general when buying olive oil, it is best to buy from retailers that let you taste the oil to ensure you enjoy it, and in small quantities, as once the container is opened, the oil deteriorates quickly. It's also better to buy two small cans or bottles than one bigger one, and avoid buying olive oil that comes in a plastic bottle, as the chemicals in plastic leak into the oil. Finally, try to buy olive oil that is less than a year old, as it will have the greatest antioxidant activity. (Look for the "pressed on" or "harvested on" date on the bottle.)

especially growing herbs, you can plant your own Mediterranean herb garden and enjoy your harvest daily. (A Mediterranean combination could include rosemary, thyme, oregano, sage, basil, marjoram, mint, tarragon, chervil, chives, and flat-leaf parsley.) But even if you don't have a green thumb, these

---

Is There a "Best" Olive?

The answer to that question is partly about what you prefer, taste-wise. I recommend that you try a variety of olives; they can be green, purple, and black, small and large, and/or with a mixture of varieties. Purchase them jarred right off the shelf, or from a specialty grocer. (Canned olives can be fine, as well, though not always as flavorful. Choose BPA-free cans.) Some supermarket salad bars now offer wonderful selections of high-quality imported olives. You can also do your own "mix"—see Marinated Mediterranean Olives and Vegetables (page 170). Just like sauerkraut, olives that come from a brine solution provide a good source of gut-friendly probiotics, plus olives provide a good source of fiber and healthy fats.

Here's the bigger issue, as far as I'm concerned: From a culinary perspective, olives with pits are much better than those that have been pitted, although this is a hard adjustment for some Americans. (Once pitted, the olives are returned to the brine for packing, which can penetrate the inside of the olive and turn it mushy and pasty, as well as increase the absorption of salt. That saltier taste can mask subtler flavors.) Some would say that without the pits, olives are a briny, soggy mess. They lose their plumpness, their flavor, and do not belong on a table with fine food. If you or your guests prefer the tidiness of eating already pitted olives, then you can still have them—just buy unpitted olives and pit them right before serving.

HERBS AND SPICES

The Basics

Like olive oil, the flavors of the Mediterranean shine through in a variety of herbs, from quintessentially Italian rosemary to distinctly French tarragon, Greek oregano, and everything in between—parsley, basil, thyme, marjoram, sage, chervil, chives, mint, and more. If you are into gardening,

days it's quite easy to locate fresh herbs in most markets—and a daily dose of herbs and spices is absolutely essential.

That's because so many of these—often grown for their medicinal properties, as well as their flavors—have anti-inflammatory and antioxidant characteristics that some researchers think contribute to the health and longevity of Mediterranean dwellers. Scientists have studied the inhabitants of

Acciaroli, Italy, a mountain village located in the Salerno region perched right above the Mediterranean. One in sixty people live to the age of 90 or older—an even better ratio than Okinawa, Sardinia, Ikaria, or any of the other Blue Zones. And they are largely free of illness, dementia, bone fractures, cataracts, and many of the other ailments that come with very old age. One thing they do every day? They use copious amounts of rosemary in their cooking, researchers have noted.

Garlic is also an herb, and an essential flavor in many Mediterranean dishes. (Many of my Mediterranean Method recipes use garlic.) This anti-inflammatory food has been shown to lower blood pressure, improve cholesterol profiles, and prevent blood clots. It contains a compound called allicin, which is released when garlic is chopped, crushed, or pressed. Allicin can be destroyed with high heat, so don't overcook your garlic! Best is to add it during the last few minutes over low heat.

Dried spices such as cinnamon, ginger, and ground chili pepper blends also offer a depth of flavor and deliver medicinal benefits, including blood sugar control. Turmeric is more typical as part of a curry-like spice mixture, but it's gaining in popularity because it contains a powerful anti-inflammatory compound known as curcumin, which is linked to improved memory, reduced arthritis symptoms, and lowering inflammation. It's not a traditional European Mediterranean flavor; it is used in the Middle East and Northern Africa, and like so many other spices, it's worth adding it to your regular rotation of daily herbs and spices!

The Extras

Fresh or dried? If you can get fresh herbs—or better yet, grow a few varieties yourself—they are superb for their taste. But of course, especially in the dead of winter, dried herbs work wonderfully. A generous sprinkle of dried herbes de Provence, fines herbes, a pinch of red pepper flakes, or a blend of Italian seasonings will always lend your food a Mediterranean accent. (For information on what herbs and spices to stock in your kitchen, see Chapter 8.)

Don't just think of herbs as accents for your food; they are food on their own. Arugula, mache, and other small greens are actually herbs packed with polyphenols. In Greece, many of the long-lived Ikaria islanders drink an herbal tea (infusion) each day made from just-gathered fresh herbs—and it's not always the same herb. Some days it may be mint tea, other days it's wild sage. You may not be able to wander along a sunny mountain path with an ocean view and gather free-growing herbs, but you can certainly do what the Ikarians do by making your own herbal teas and infusions. (For a simple tea, place a handful of fresh herbs of your choice in a cup, cover with water that you brought to a boil, let steep, strain, and drink. For more on herbal infusions and teas, see page 41.)

YOGURT AND/OR KEFIR:
1 serving = 6–8 ounces

The Basics

Yogurt is a fermented milk product, as is its less famous cousin kefir, a yogurt-style drink. Both of these probiotic foods contain live and active bacteria such as *Lactobacillus acidophilus*. If you tolerate dairy, you can have them daily. If you are dairy intolerant, or you simply avoid dairy products, then aim to consume non-dairy yogurt options made from nut milks instead.

The yogurt sections in many supermarkets are minefields of "yogurt products" loaded with sugar, artificial flavorings, and other additives; what they may not have are the live active cultures that make it a great probiotic pick. Avoid processed yogurt products and stick with plain, organic yogurt from pasture-raised animals. Go Greek—as in Greek-style yogurt—for its generally higher protein content, though regular yogurt is higher in calcium. (These differences are due to how these two styles of yogurt are made; Greek yogurt involves straining out the extra liquid in regular yogurt.)

The Extras

At its best, yogurt is farm-fresh, unprocessed, and plain, meant to be eaten with fresh fruit and/or perhaps a small drizzle (½ teaspoon) of local honey. Because yogurt (and kefir) are increasingly popular, it's fairly easy to find organic plain (unflavored) varieties in most large supermarkets. But even kefir—once obscure—has now been "Americanized"— with sugary, flavored versions popping up. As with yogurt, pick pure and plain! Blend with berries for a smoothie, and use it in place of plain yogurt in dips and dressings.

DARK CHOCOLATE:
1 serving = 1–2 ounces

The Basics

I love to tell my patients that they can—they *should*—eat a bit of dark chocolate every day! (Few of us would refuse chocolate, after all.) But . . . it should *always* be dark chocolate—least 74 to 80 percent cacao. Dark chocolate has anti-inflammatory flavonoids that contribute to brain and heart health, and is associated with a lowered risk for diabetes. It is also a great source of prebiotic fiber and helps support healthy gut bacteria. Milk chocolate and white chocolate, however, have a higher sugar content that you (and your blood sugar) should avoid. The Italians, French, and Spanish love chocolate and produce some exquisite varieties of dark chocolate. I don't know that they eat it every day, but everyone should do so, based on what we know about its benefits.

The Extras

A 1- to 2-ounce serving of dark chocolate is roughly ¼ to ⅓ of a typical chocolate bar (read the label for net weight)—not a hardship for most of us who love chocolate! But if you want to enjoy it another way, melt it over fresh fruit. You can also add 1 tablespoon of cocoa powder to your morning coffee and drink your chocolate serving. (Whisk the cocoa with a bit of boiling water before adding to your coffee, if you are concerned that it won't dissolve entirely.) When shopping for cocoa, choose "natural" or "non-alkalized" for maximum flavonoids; Dutch processing, which is done to improve flavor and lower acidity, unfortunately lowers flavonoid content.

RED WINE:
1–2 (5-ounce) servings for women/
2–3 (5-ounce) servings for men

The Basics

Red wine to complement your food is a traditional part of a true Mediterranean meal—and it yields some of the powerful health benefits of this diet. We know that moderate alcohol consumption is associated with positive brain and heart health, in part because it functions as an anti-inflammatory. (And overconsumption of alcohol is, of course, associated with elevated health risks, including cancer—discussed in Chapter 7.) But red wine, by far, is the alcohol that offers the most neuroprotective and cardiovascular benefits, and the lowest cancer risk as well. Red wine is also made and produced throughout the Mediterranean. There are numerous white wines and rosés from the region—but red wine consistently emerges from the research as the healthiest pick, as the skins of red wine grapes have more polyphenols (antioxidants) than white wine grapes, including the polyphenol resveratrol.

On the Italian island of Sardinia, a Blue Zone, there are large concentrations of people who live past the age of 100. Sardinians famously drink an everyday red wine made from the dark purple Cannonau grape grown all over the island, and it is particularly rich in beneficial polyphenols—more so than red wine grapes from neighboring countries such as France, Spain, and even mainland Italy. Cannonau was once thought to be the exact same as the Garnacha (or, more commonly, Grenache) grape that originated in Spain (and is one of the most widely planted grape varieties in the world). However, archaeologists

have found preserved grape seeds on Sardinia that are more than 3,000 years old. The seeds' DNA indicates a difference from today's Grenache and its cousins, implying that this particular Mediterranean wine, with its higher resveratrol content, is indeed special—and perhaps responsible for the number of healthy and long-lived Sardinians. (That said, and to the dismay of proud Sardinians, most people still refer to Cannonau as Grenache.)

The right wine is good for your health—but in the right quantities, which is to say, in moderation: no more than two to three 5-ounce servings per day with food. Because of how men and women metabolize alcohol differently (due in part to hormones, as well as body mass), recommended servings for women are slightly fewer (1 to 2 glasses). Women metabolize alcohol more slowly due to the presence of estrogen and progesterone; for that reason, if a woman and man of the same size drink the same amount of alcohol, her blood alcohol level will be higher for a longer period of time.

The Extras

Any red wine has benefit when consumed in moderation and with meals, including blends, cabernets, merlots, pinot noirs, and many other varieties. You can find inexpensive domestic and imported wines throughout the United States. Choose any red that you like, whether it's Old World wine (from mostly European wine-producing regions) or New World (including South America, Australia, New Zealand, and the U.S.). Pick what you enjoy and can afford. More expensive wines are not necessarily better for your health, although there is likely some health benefit to organic wines.

Beyond picking red wine, consider dry farm wines when available, as well. Dry farm wines—wines that don't use irrigation—have less sugar content and slightly less alcohol than wines produced with irrigation. Vintners who avoid irrigation in general also use fewer pesticides and herbicides. For help finding these health-conscious vintners, visit www.drmasley.com/resources.

I am not pushing nondrinkers to start drinking alcohol, as you may have a very good reason for avoiding it. But if you do drink alcohol in moderation, then I recommend that you consume mostly red wine.

If you can't limit yourself to 2 to 3 servings per day and usually end up drinking more, then please do not drink alcohol at all. Excess alcohol intake isn't just terrible for your health; it can also ruin your life, impacting your relationship with family and loved ones, and worsen your job performance, as well.

Even without red wine, if you're still eating a broad range of healthy foods on the Mediterranean diet, you'll get most of the benefits. To maximize your health gains, do make sure to add red-purple plant pigments that offer similar antioxidant compounds as red wine—try berries, cherries, red grapes, and blueberries, and eat them every day.

COFFEE:
1–2 servings/Tea: 3–4 servings per day

The Basics

Like many Americans, Mediterranean dwellers love their daily coffee. In the morning, it's usually a strong espresso or two—and if you are served a morning cappuccino, a café con leche, or a café au lait, they bear no resemblance to the sugar-packed "coffee drinks," sweetened with flavored syrups and topped with whipped cream, that you'll find in the United States. Whether you prefer regular coffee, espresso, or tea, the helpful ingredients here are the pigments in coffee and tea (flavonoids and catechins). Caffeine intake is also associated with a boost in cognitive function and even lower rates of depression, but even decaf versions have health benefits from the flavonoid pigments.

The caffeine content from coffee varies based on the source/roaster/brand, but even taking that into account, people who are caffeine sensitive should have 1, but not more than 2, servings of coffee per day (more is harmful and increases the risk for cardiovascular events). People who are not caffeine sensitive benefit from having 2 to 3 servings of coffee per day, but again, more is harmful. It's healthiest if you drink it black. Though you can add a touch of organic milk or half-and-half (or a non-dairy alternative), don't add sugar or sweeteners or you'll cancel out the health benefits of drinking coffee.

Not everyone likes coffee, and if you don't drink it now, don't feel compelled to start. If you're a tea drinker, you can get even more benefits from consuming black or green tea than you do from coffee. You'll have to drink a bit more—the average cup of coffee has 60 mg of caffeine and the average cup of tea has between 25 and 35 mg. Tea drinkers who are caffeine sensitive can have 2 to 4 servings per day, but for those who aren't, 3 to 6 servings per day of tea is fine.

And not everyone likes caffeine, either, or can tolerate it. If you feel better caffeine-free, go for decaffeinated teas and coffees if you like. Decaf tea has L-theanine (see below) and decaf coffee has flavonoid pigments.

The Extras

Green tea offers a compound called L-theanine, a brain-boosting amino acid. The problem with regular green tea is that when you toss the tea bag, you're also tossing the antioxidants and L-theanine. That's why powdered matcha tea is superior, because when combined with boiling water, those compounds will dissolve into the liquid that you consume. Matcha green tea isn't from the Mediterranean; it is a product of Japan, and the Blue Zone Okinawans enjoy it daily, and you likely should, too.

One 1-ounce serving of espresso, contrary to popular belief, doesn't deliver more caffeine to your system than the typical 8-ounce cup of coffee, but that's because it's a much smaller beverage. Ounce per ounce, espresso is considerably more caffeinated; on average, espresso has 25 to 35 mg of caffeine per ounce, while regular coffee can have as few as 8 mg per ounce. (A reminder here, though, that caffeine quantities can vary based on brand.) That's something to keep in mind if you like to have more than one espresso in a sitting, or you regularly drink double espressos.

If you regularly consume both caffeinated coffee and tea over the course of your day, keep tabs on how much you're having, since it can be easy to overdo caffeine, especially later in the day when it could interfere with your sleep. I suggest no more than 2 cups of coffee and 2 cups of tea; any additional beverages should be decaf.

The real benefits are coming from the plant pigments, not the caffeine. And whether you choose coffee or tea, regular or decaf, feel free to do something that's still considered more American than Mediterranean (despite their hot summers): Pour it over ice and enjoy.

WATER

The Basics

Do you need to follow the oft-repeated "8 glasses of water a day" rule? Maybe not, if you're drinking other fluids and eating an abundance of vegetables and fruits that hold water, but you should consume plenty of water over the course of your day. If you feel thirsty, that is a tad late, as you are already dehydrated. Your body needs fluids! (Unfortunately, as we age our sense of thirst is diminished.) Your daily consumption of coffee and tea can count toward your regular hydration, but the caffeine in coffee, in particular, is a diuretic, so make sure you replenish your fluids with some water throughout the day.

Drinking mineral water with meals is a common tradition in the Mediterranean. Grocery stores throughout the region devote tremendous amounts of shelf space to bottled waters, with many brands touting their mineral content, their origin, or even their medical and digestive benefits. Feel free to enjoy flat or sparkling mineral water, if you like, not so much for the minerals as because it's a nice upgrade from tap water!

To ensure your home drinking water is clean and chemical free, I do recommend having a reverse-osmosis filter at the kitchen sink for drinking water and cooking. It will also screen out inorganic copper (a potential brain toxin) associated with copper pipes. For details on inorganic copper see page 107 in Chapter 5.

The Extras

Here's another Mediterranean tradition that you can adopt: Hydrate with homemade herbal infusions and teas. Use a variety of herbal combinations that appeal to you. Peppermint, verbena, and chamomile are common, but experiment with other herbs such as rosemary, sage, thyme, and oregano. Add 2 to 3 tablespoons of fresh herbs to 1 cup of hot water, allow to steep for 2 to 3 minutes, then drink hot or refrigerate and enjoy cold. You can also put fresh herbs into a glass pitcher, cover, and "brew" outside in the sun for several hours.

Wait, Where's the Pasta?

THE EVERYDAY ESSENTIALS outlined here are the foundation you'll build on going forward. The foods we're about to discuss, which you should have several times a week, will fill out your plate and give you even more menu options and inspiration in the kitchen. But, you may be wondering, what about grains? What about bread and pasta? Aren't those daily Mediterranean mainstays?

While they are foods you'll find in that region, most of the benefit of the Mediterranean diet comes from eating more vegetables, fruits, beans, nuts, olive oil, and other healthy fats, as well as reducing red meat and having moderate amounts of red wine with meals—not from eating whole grains and cereals, which provided minimal benefits. This was the conclusion of a highly regarded study (the 2012 EPIC Greek Cohort study, discussed in Chapter 4, for its conclusions on heart health) that tracked almost 24,000 Greek citizens for years, analyzing each component of their diet in an attempt to understand what food groups provided the most overall benefits to health, disease prevention, and longevity. Furthermore, while the fiber in whole grains was beneficial, the overall glycemic load of grains—the sugar load delivered into the bloodstream, a point we'll dive into in a moment—was not.

In the United States, one of our "Mediterranean misfires" is to help ourselves to generous amounts of pasta and bread, or to use a bowl of whole grains as the basis for a meal. But there's a problem and it's not just a misfire—it's a mismatch. We can't adopt this way of eating and call it healthy when other aspects of our American lifestyle—including our level of physical activity—are so different. Most of us struggle to get more than seven hours of exercise per week. A Spanish fisherman, a French shepherd, or an Italian farmer who goes home and eats a dinner that includes grains—rice, couscous, pasta, polenta, bread—has earned such a meal because he's active seven-plus hours a *day*. And even they likely have a much smaller portion of grains than we serve regularly in the United States.

Soaking up that rich tomato sauce from your pasta dinner with a piece of bread is tempting. The Italians even have a name for it: *fare la scarpetta*, or to "make a little shoe" (as in the shape of the bread used to scrape your plate clean). But if you're doing it all the time, it won't make you healthier or thinner—in fact, it's just the opposite, because your level of physical activity is likely way too low, even if you work out.

The answer, you may be thinking, is to be more active—*lots* more active. That's partly true. Depending on your activity level, you may be able to have whole grains and pasta a few times a week, and you don't need to be training for the Tour de France to get there.

However, there is another factor to consider: how flour products—even whole grains—behave in your body. And for most of us, they behave just like sugar. If one pillar of the Mediterranean diet is to *choose fresh, whole foods like the everyday essentials* just mentioned, the other equally important one—and the one that makes my Mediterranean Method so effective—is to *choose foods that will keep your blood sugar in balance*, which is the key to staying healthy and trim, as well as reducing your risk of chronic disease. Fortunately, with this style of eating, that's simple to do.

Choose Foods with a Low Glycemic Load

MOST FOODS HAVE the ability to elevate your blood sugar and contain some level of a *glycemic load*: a reference to how high a person's blood sugar goes after consuming a standard "real world" serving of a particular carbohydrate food.* Foods can be categorized as

---

* Note: This is different from the glycemic "index," which has been misused. It calculates values based on 50 grams of carb load from any food, whether it's a vegetable, a grain, an animal product, or other. Here's a favorite example: 50 grams of carbs from carrots—about 9 large carrots—has a "high" glycemic index and 50 grams of carbs from white-flour pasta—a scant cup—is "moderate." Someone could conclude that pasta is less "sugary" and therefore healthier than

high, medium, or low in their glycemic load. You won't be surprised that eating a high-glycemic-load food like a candy bar sends your blood sugar soaring (and then crashing). So will a glass of orange juice, a bagel, or a bowl of white rice—or even a bag of salty pretzels! All of them are high-glycemic-load carbohydrates that essentially dump sugars into your system very quickly—just the opposite of "slow-release" carbs such as high-fiber vegetables or beans.

Poor blood sugar control is the cause of a host of health issues. The shortlist includes obesity, heart disease, diabetes, metabolic syndrome (a dangerous combination of risk factors for heart disease and diabetes), dementia, and Alzheimer's disease. But there is a simple fix that doesn't involve years of medication or surgical interventions: Change your dietary habits and choose a low-glycemic Mediterranean style of eating—the Mediterranean Method. (Note: If you're curious, skip ahead to the glycemic-load tables at the end of Chapter 8 to see what common foods—including those on a Mediterranean diet—are classified as low, medium, and high.)

Foods to Eat Several Times a Week

Fish and seafood, poultry, eggs, whole grains, probiotic-rich dairy (including cheese)

Now that you have an understanding of the importance of choosing low-glycemic-load foods for controlling your blood sugar (a key Mediterranean Method concept we'll revisit in the health chapters to come), the rest of the foods that constitute the Mediterranean diet will make even more sense—as will the frequency of how often you should have them.

These aren't daily must-haves but, rather, foods you can add several days of the week to round out your meals and give you more choices.

Among these options are animal proteins, and as you'll see it's important to *choose "clean" protein*, not *"mean" protein*—from animals raised without pesticide-loaded grains or antibiotics, or growth hormones. Factory-farmed, feedlot animals come to mind regarding the latter, but it's not just poultry or

carrots. But no one eats 9 carrots in one sitting, and most people consume more than 1 cup of pasta. The index is not a good tool for everyday use by nonprofessionals; it's easy to misapply the data. (In reality, one typical serving of carrots has a low sugar load, and one serving of pasta has a high sugar load, showing the importance of using a food's glycemic load, not its glycemic index.)

other meat at issue. The eggs, milk, yogurt, cheese, and butter you consume should come from organic-fed, cage-free, and pasture-raised animals as much as possible.

This isn't simply for humane, environmental reasons, though those are numerous; it's because toxic herbicides, pesticides, antibiotics, hormones, and other chemical substances eventually make their way into *your* body when you consume food products made from animals that ingest them. Whether it's the chicken you eat for dinner, the eggs at breakfast, or the yogurt you snack on, residues of these compounds are particularly concentrated in saturated fats, and we know they are harmful to human health, as they have been linked to diseases ranging from cancer and diabetes to Alzheimer's. Glyphosate, the active ingredient in the herbicide Roundup, is a probable human carcinogen, but it's still widely used, allowing grazing animals to ingest it. Growth hormones don't just fatten up animals; they make us fat, too.

You do pay more for foods from animals that aren't part of an industrial-scale operation, but ultimately it's about your health and longevity, and those of anyone else who eats at your table. If you cannot access organic animal products, keep in mind that because toxins linger in animal fat, you can avoid some of these harmful substances if you pick low-fat options—use chicken breast, not thighs with skin, for instance, or make an egg-white-only omelet, as the yolks are the magnet for the substances you want to avoid, or a lean sirloin steak instead of prime rib. If you can't find clean, eat lean.

FISH AND SEAFOOD:
3–5 times per week

The Basics

Most Americans overlook a key source of dietary protein—one that offers brain-boosting, heart-healthy benefits: fish and other seafood, including seaweed. This should be a part of your meal three to five times per week. There are many reasons why some people shy away from seafood: . . . *It's too expensive . . . I don't know how to prepare it . . . I don't like it . . . What about mercury?* But seafood is a main component of a Mediterranean diet—it's a coastal region, after all—and it's a foundational food among the Japanese, including Blue Zone Okinawans who have such low rates of chronic disease.

Cold-water fish, shellfish, and seaweed contain high levels of long-chain omega-3 fatty acids, strongly linked to brain and heart health but an essential fatty acid our bodies cannot produce on their own. Therefore, we must get them from food (or supplements—see page 87), and seafood happens to be an excellent dietary source.

Research shows that we obtain the most heart and brain benefits from omega-3 fats through eating fish. But what if you don't eat fish? If you are vegetarian, then consume seaweed (as a salad) three to five times per week, or take a DHA seaweed supplement. And if you truly don't like the taste of any type of seafood, including fish and seaweed, supplement with a high-quality fish oil (and high-quality is key—see page 87 for more information). Some experts recommend walnuts, flax seed, and other plants as omega-3 sources, but these are medium-chain fats, not long-chain; they are healthy, to be sure, but these fats don't deliver the same protective benefits as the omega-3s found in seafood.

Finally, remember that the "clean protein" rule isn't limited to land animals. Farmed fish, including salmon raised in large-scale industrial conditions, ingest pesticide-contaminated feed, too. You'll avoid that issue with wild-caught, responsibly sourced fish; if the fish you buy is farmed, ideally you should know where it was produced (was the water clean?) and what it was fed, but in reality these features are very difficult to determine. A good source of information on this topic is the Environmental Defense Fund's Seafood Selector.

The Extras

Once you're ready to dive in, what kind of fish should you choose? The type of fish you bring home from the market is actually more important than how often you eat it, as you're after those valuable omega-3 fatty acids. Two of the very best sources are salmon and sardines, both cold-water, fatty fish with high concentrations of omega-3s, though other varieties such as mussels and trout (plus more varieties I'll discuss later) are also good picks.

While sardines are popular throughout countries along the Mediterranean Sea, salmon is a fish we tend to associate with the Pacific Northwest, including Alaska and British Columbia, although you'll see Atlantic salmon from northern Europe on many menus in Mediterranean countries.

Plankton and algae (unlike humans) produce their own omega-3 fats, which they must do to thrive in cold water. Small fish eat the plankton and algae and store their omega-3s; those small fish in turn are eaten by larger ones, further concentrating this essential fatty

acid. The colder the water and the higher the fish is on the food chain, the higher its omega-3 content. But, though larger fish may have more omega-3 content, be careful with extra-large varieties like swordfish and tuna. These wide-mouth fish are the ones with the highest concentrations of something you want to steer clear of: mercury. Mercury occurs in tiny amounts in plankton, so the more plankton and smaller plankton-eating fish the extra-large fish consume, the more mercury they will accumulate in their bodies. Tuna shows up in many traditional Mediterranean recipes, but I don't recommend it to all my patients because of mercury concerns. (You can substitute canned salmon for most recipes where you'd use canned tuna.)

Don't be concerned about choosing "authentic" Mediterranean fish, unless you're lucky enough to be living in the region for the season and visiting the local fish markets in the morning. Wherever you are, buy what is fresh and avoid or at least limit the large-mouth fish species (tuna, grouper, bass, king fish, shark, and swordfish). If you can't find quality fresh fish in your part of the country, consider paying a bit more and order some high-quality, vacuum-packed seafood. Often, flash-frozen and individually vacuum-packed fish is the best quality and the least fishy—sometimes better than fresh. The emphasis here, though, has to be on freshly caught fish that is vacuum packed and flash-frozen. (See the resource section at www.drmasley.com /resources for my favorite sources for vacuum-packed, flash-frozen fish.) White fish—such as the omnipresent tilapia, cod, or catfish—are fine, but they aren't my first preference as they're considerably lower in omega-3s than salmon, sardines, anchovies, herring, mussels, oysters, squid, octopus, sole/flounder, and trout.

POULTRY:
3–5 times per week

The Basics

Poultry isn't as obvious a choice in Mediterranean cuisine as seafood, but it's still popular because it's inexpensive and it's easy to find in most markets, where it's usually organic and fresh, and more flavorful—very different from the factory-farmed poultry raised with antibiotics, pesticide-loaded grains, and growth hormones that most American shoppers see in their supermarkets.

Unlike seafood, poultry doesn't offer the benefits of omega-3 fatty acids. (In the EPIC Greek Cohort study, including poultry in one's diet did not have the clear health benefits of other foods, but it can still be a clean and lean, versatile protein source. Choose organically raised chicken, turkey, and duck.)

The Extras

You can easily give poultry a Mediterranean twist with the right herbs and spices. For example, make a paste of chopped garlic, rosemary, sea salt, lemon juice and zest, and a bit of virgin olive oil, and spread it over chicken breasts or thighs. Let them marinate in the refrigerator for an hour or more, then grill or cook as desired. You can do this with any combination of herbs and garlic, but lemon has a way of really bringing out the flavor. Try Moroccan Spiced Chicken (page 202) for a North African–inspired dish, or if you want a switch from chicken, make Duck with Port Wine Sauce and Mashed

Sweet Potato (page 203) or Mediterranean Turkey Stew (page 205).

EGGS: 1 SERVING =
1–2 eggs, 3–5 times/week

The Basics

Like poultry, eggs aren't necessarily a daily go-to food in the Mediterranean region, but they are used as an inexpensive and always-available protein source, in delicious ways, and they don't just show up at breakfast. In Spain, you'll find a crisp and savory "tortilla" made with eggs, potatoes, and vegetables. French soufflés and quiches rely on eggs, as do Italian frittatas and salads. Try the Mediterranean Wild Mushroom Omelet (page 164), the Frittata with Spinach, Mushrooms, and Cheese (page 166), the Spanish Tortilla (page 209), or the Salade Niçoise (page 182).

The Extras

As with poultry, choose organic and cage-free eggs.

The vast majority of research regarding egg consumption in the last five to ten years has shown that eating eggs does not raise cholesterol levels, and most scientists have suggested that moderate egg consumption will not increase the risk for heart disease. However, the debate has not ended, and at least one recent study has suggested that egg consumption and the saturated fat that comes with it may increase the risk for cardiovascular events and shorten overall life span. This controversy will likely continue.

The biggest concern is not that eggs have a modest amount of saturated fat, which is all in the egg yolk. A more alarming issue is that commercially raised eggs are loaded with pesticides and other chemicals. I have always recommended that if my patients eat products with egg yolks, they buy organically raised, cage-free eggs.

I've also advised my patients with known heart disease, or multiple cardiovascular risk factors, to keep their saturated-fat intake modest, not excessive, which certainly would allow for eggs to be served three to five times per week, especially when following my form of a Mediterranean diet that otherwise has very little saturated fat.

WHOLE GRAINS:
3–5 times per week (depending on activity level)

The Basics

Many people rely on grains and cereals (including whole grains) for "heart-healthy" fiber. However, given their significant glycemic loads and impact on blood sugar, for most people, even whole grains should be limited to a few times per week. In addition, paying attention to portion size as it relates to your level of physical activity is important. If you're trying to lose weight, those factors become even more critical. (See page 73.)

If you're struggling to get more than 7 hours of exercise per week, limit your whole-grain consumption to ½ to ⅔ cup, three or four times per week. If you are more active, you can likely tolerate having 1 cup of whole grains per day. If you're extremely active—that is, you have a truly physically-taxing job or you're an athlete—then you can have more. (Note: These are cooked amounts. So, 2 ounces of uncooked whole-grain pasta,

rice, or other grain/cereal usually yields about 1 cup cooked, but check the labels.)

Regarding pasta portions, here is where we have expanded upon the European portion in a big way. Order pasta with marinara sauce in Italy, and you'll likely get a pasta portion that covers a small salad plate, covered with a delightful marinara sauce, and after this little morsel, then you'll go on and eat the main course with some form of protein, a large portion of vegetables, and some beans on the side. In the United States, the standard is to cook 2 ounces of dried pasta per person, which provides 4.5 ounces of cooked pasta (and people often eat double this portion size, served on an extra-large plate). In Italy, though, you'd probably be fed 1 to 2 ounces of *cooked* pasta; so, Americans are eating double or quadruple the Italian portion. See Spaghetti with Marinara Sauce and Mushrooms (page 173) as an appetizer for an example of an appropriate portion size.

The Extras

Though many Mediterranean dwellers eat grains, research such as the EPIC study shows that most benefits from this diet are coming from other food groups, most notably vegetables and fruits, olive oil, and red wine, as well as from foods they *don't* eat, including processed foods, high-sugar foods, red meat, and junk food. Certainly fiber is essential, but to maintain balanced blood sugar—and avoid all the metabolic problems associated with blood sugar fluctuations—get most of your fiber from vegetables, fruits, beans, nuts, and dark chocolate, rather than from whole grains, including whole-grain breads.

Perhaps you're thinking that you can get around the high glycemic load of grains and cereals by exchanging white-flour products for whole-grain ones. Whole-grain flour does have more nutrients than white flour, but as soon as *any* grain is ground up and pulverized into flour, it behaves like sugar in your body. Whole-wheat bread falls into this category. (For more on flour products, see pages 51–52; for more on bread, as well as gluten, see pages 120–125.)

Here's a general look at where most grains and cereals, including whole grains, rank in terms of their glycemic load.

High

- White pasta/macaroni/noodles
- Rice (including risotto), brown, white, basmati
- Corn (including polenta)
- Most quick-cooking/instant grains (boxed couscous or pilaf mixes)

Medium

- Whole-grain pastas (especially protein-enriched pasta)
- Wild rice
- Pearled barley
- Oats/oatmeal
- Quinoa
- Tabbouleh (bulgur)
- Farro (wheat)

Low

- Steel-cut oats

It is possible to slow down the quick-release impact of grains when you combine them with plenty of fiber, protein, and smart fat. For example, instead of having white pasta, try whole-grain pasta with mixed roasted vegetables, white beans, and baby spinach tossed with extra-virgin olive oil. Or, even better, enjoy protein- and fiber-enriched pasta that is made with garbanzo bean flour. Barilla (the Italian pasta company) has created an excellent pasta with added garbanzo bean flour that has 42 percent lower glycemic load than regular pasta. Add some lean protein like chicken or half a portion of seafood on the side, and it becomes a complete meal. Less than 1 cup of whole grains may seem meager, but when combined with other ingredients such as those—which is also Mediterranean style—they become more filling, satisfying, and nutrient-dense.

For a discussion on what to eat for breakfast on a Mediterranean diet—particularly if you've been relying on foods like cereals and toast and other bread products—see pages 163–168. (As you can see from the list, oatmeal and steel-cut oats are possible options; don't forget eggs—just discussed—and read on for more about dairy choices, such as yogurt.)

PROBIOTIC-RICH DAIRY, INCLUDING CHEESE:
3–5 times a week or more

The Basics

Probiotic foods, which naturally contain living organisms such as bacteria and yeasts, promote the growth of "good" gut bacteria that contribute to your overall health, and can ultimately help to keep blood sugar levels balanced. While you can take probiotic supplements to keep these beneficial microbes going strong, there are some excellent dietary sources of probiotics that fit into the Mediterranean diet, including some cheeses and yogurt and kefir. (See page 36 for information on yogurt and kefir, which can be eaten daily, or at least three to five times per week.)

Raw cheeses, so termed because they are made with raw, unpasteurized milk (cow, sheep, or goat), are good examples of probiotic-rich dairy foods. (The heat used in pasteurization destroys the milk's bacteria—and therefore the probiotic qualities of the dairy product.) There are many varieties of raw-milk cheese, from Parmigiano Reggiano, to French camembert, to aged cheddars.

For some individuals, raw, unpasteurized dairy products may be dangerous to consume, particularly for anyone with a compromised immune system. For most healthy people, at least in Europe, they are considered generally safe. Furthermore, owing to strict rules governing the sale of raw-milk cheeses in the United States, any cheese made from unpasteurized milk must be aged a minimum of 60 days, which is considered enough time for the salts and acids in the cheese to destroy harmful bacteria such as listeria, salmonella, and *E. coli*. Still, check with your health-care provider if you stand to benefit, or if you face more risk, from adding raw-milk cheeses and unpasteurized dairy to your diet, and follow the provider's advice.

If you don't eat dairy products, you'll find other sources of probiotic foods in Chapter 6, as well as information on how to choose probiotic supplements.

The Extras

Europeans along the Mediterranean (and throughout the continent, for that matter) take their cheese very seriously! (One bite of an authentic French reblochon, comte, or camembert, and you'll wonder what that stuff is that you've been eating back in the U.S.)

Besides knowing their way around a wheel of cheese—probiotic or not—Europeans also know that moderation is key, particularly because cheese is a high-saturated fat, a rich food. A small portion of good-quality cheese lends a depth of flavor to a dish, but it's not an overwhelming presence. On its own, it's a small but savory treat, perhaps after dinner, served with nuts and fruit. Typically, the serving size for cheese is not more than 1 ounce. Or, to put it more plainly, here are some cheesy foods you won't find on a Mediterranean diet (besides a slice of American cheese): cheeseburgers, nachos, fried mozzarella sticks, anything buried under a blanket of melted cheese . . . you get the idea.

Of course, not all dairy is probiotic-rich—that really only applies to raw cheeses, yogurt, and kefir, not to milk, cream, or butter. On a Mediterranean diet, butter (in particular clarified butter, also called ghee) might be used sparingly, but the fat of choice is olive oil. Limit the consumption of butter, cream, and other high-fat dairy items in favor of olive oil, and always choose organic products from pastured animals.

Occasional Foods

Red meat, flour products (bread and pasta), potatoes, sweets

Finally, here are some foods that are naturally limited on the Mediterranean diet—items that aren't usually included in meals because they aren't a traditional part of the regional cuisine or because they are viewed as treats. (There are also items such as flour products that should be limited because of their high glycemic load.)

To maximize the disease-preventive benefits of the Mediterranean way of eating, limit occasional foods to no more than once or twice a week, if you choose to eat them at all. You'll notice you won't find "recommended servings" next to these foods, because you should not consider them essential. Enjoy them if you want to, but approach them as once-in-a-while foods.

This "special occasions" mindset is a lesson worth bringing back home. Studies show that while the Mediterranean diet is important for what it includes, it's probable that many people who follow this plan have lower rates of heart disease, diabetes, neurodegenerative diseases, gut problems, cancer, and other health problems because of what they *don't* eat.

For generations, red meat was historically more expensive and not as easy to source as seafood, so it was used sparingly. Sweets were also more costly and therefore were reserved for celebrations. But even after such foods became more affordable and available,

the old ways have persisted. The healthiest Mediterranean dwellers have naturally avoided overconsumption of two foods that average Americans eat every day.

We'd do best, and probably live longer, if we adopted this save-it-for-a-special-occasion approach when planning our meals. Celebrating with food is part of life. Why not make it a long and healthy one?

RED MEAT

The Basics

If you eat red meat, choosing clean protein is essential. As discussed, feedlot animals that eat pesticide-coated grain or hay treated with herbicides and pesticides, and who ingest (or are injected with) growth hormones, will then pass those toxins on to you. You are what you eat, so don't eat dirty protein.

In addition to how animals are raised, there is the issue of how the meat is processed. Nitrosamines are preservatives used in the preparation of cured meats such as deli meats, bacon, sausage, and ham—and they are also linked to cancer, insulin resistance, and cognitive decline. This is another reason to choose organic and pasture-raised products; check the labels to make sure they are labeled "nitrate-free" or "nitrosamine-free" so that you don't ingest these chemicals.

The Extras

In the Mediterranean, red meat is eaten as a main course only a few times per month, and in a 4- to 5-ounce portion. It's not that it's prohibitively expensive; it's that it's not typical of coastal regions. In a seaside town, if it's not primarily seafood on the menu, you'll likely find more poultry (or pork, lamb, and rabbit) than you will beef. Farther inland throughout the Mediterranean basin, you will find more red meat, but it's still not eaten daily or in enormous amounts, and it's usually fresh and pasture-raised. *Cucina povera*—food of the poor—is an Italian phrase, but virtually every country has some version of this approach to being frugal with more precious items like meat, and rounding things out with what was easily available from one's garden or farm—inexpensive staples like dried beans, or a bit of leftover vegetables and grains from a previous meal. It's food of the poor but also, as it turns out in the Mediterranean, food of the healthy.

You may be wondering if the world-renowned cured meats from Spain, Italy, and France fall into the same risky category as preservative-laden American bacon, hot dogs, and luncheon meats. The *highest-quality*, imported jamon, prosciutto, jambon, and related products are usually free of nitrosamines, as they are produced with as much care and pride as handmade cheeses and wines. (The same cannot be said of mass-produced products.) But of course, you can ask and look at labels. Just keep in mind that these are invariably high-sodium items, so it's best to follow tradition and limit their consumption to no more than once a week.

Even though Spain has a famous string of restaurants called Museo de Jamon (yes, "Museum of Ham"), in the Mediterranean diet, cured meats and sausages are not the sole focus of a meal. Instead, they're sliced ultra-thin, served in a small portion as an appetizer with lots of other foods, and used as flavorings.

FLOUR PRODUCTS

The Basics

You are aware, now, of the high glycemic load of grain products—including whole grains (see pages 47–48), so where does that leave you with regard to bread? The fact is that white-flour bread (as well as crackers, cookies, bagels, pretzels, cake, and other flour and bread products) will send your blood sugar upward, as if you were eating table sugar.

Even whole-grain breads, a slight improvement because they have more nutrients, will do this, as their glycemic loads aren't that different from white-flour breads. As mentioned earlier, when any grain is ground into flour, its impact on your blood sugar becomes more extreme. Unless you exercise 2 to 3 hours per day, think of whole-grain bread like cake—not a daily staple, but an occasional food, once or twice a week. If you're more active, you can have it more often. I can't think of any good reason to consume any processed white-flour products, which offer zero nutritional benefits. They won't keep you healthy or trim, and if you have issues with gluten, they'll make you sick. (For information on gluten sensitivity and intolerance, see pages 120–122.) What's the only thing you *won't* get if you cut your consumption of flour products? Empty calories and high blood sugar.

The Extras

Are flour products part of the Mediterranean diet? In big, modern European grocery store chains you'll find plenty of the same unhealthy packaged cookies and crackers—complete with trans fats—that fill the aisles of American supermarkets. But those products never were and never will be part of the traditional Mediterranean diet.

Still, Europeans do eat bread. They just eat it differently. It's true that small, local bakeries all over Europe and throughout the Mediterranean turn out just-baked loaves of "daily bread" and other fresh items that people snap up in the morning or on their way home from work or school. But this is where lifestyle differences really come into play, starting with how much more active Mediterranean people tend to be than Americans. First, chances are they've walked to that corner bakery or ridden a bicycle, and that is not the only exercise they're getting over the course of their day.

Second, the quality of the bread is worth noting if it comes from a small-scale vendor. It is fresh and baked right there, not made in a factory from grain grown with chemicals, and produced with shelf-stabilizing artificial ingredients or unhealthy fats. It isn't made with preservatives and isn't sealed in a plastic bag. Instead, it's meant to be eaten that day—by tomorrow, it will be hard like a brick and nearly inedible.

The bread is also meant to be shared with others, and eaten in modest proportion to the rest of a varied and flavorful meal. You won't find a "bottomless bread basket" in a Mediterranean home. As with so many other foods, a family or a group of friends will share their bread, and eat it mindfully and joyfully.

POTATOES

The Basics

Like flour, potatoes—especially when they are baked and mashed—behave like sugar in your body. Because of their high glycemic load, view them as a once-in-a-while food.

Some experts suggest that we should consume potatoes for their "resistant starch"—a kind of starch you can't digest. Because resistant starch passes through your intestinal tract without being absorbed, your gut bacteria feed on it, breaking it down and fermenting it into short-chain fatty acids that ultimately support good gut health.

Still, there is the problematic issue of glycemic load, but those who recommend the resistant starch in potatoes for gut health also suggest there is a way to lower their high sugar load—through first cooking and then chilling the potatoes. Without delving too deeply into the biochemistry of food, here is the main idea: Chilling the cooked potatoes changes the structure of the starch, whether you eat the potatoes chilled right then, or chill them and reheat them later. Once cooked and then chilled, the potatoes have a 20 to 25 percent lower glycemic load than still-warm potatoes, and the chilled potatoes have higher levels of beneficial resistant starch, too. Whole boiled potatoes have a lower glycemic load than baked or mashed. So, if you're going to eat potatoes, boil them, then chill them in the refrigerator and serve them cold (as in a potato salad), or chill them and then heat them to serve later. And eat them whole rather than mashed.

Small, skin-on potatoes—especially red- and purple-skinned, which have more resistant starch and lower glycemic loads—are better choices than larger waxy white and russet potatoes. Sweet potatoes also have a lower glycemic load. Eating potatoes with protein and a smart fat can also lower their glycemic load.

But even if you take all the right steps and only eat small boiled potatoes that were refrigerated, they will still have a high glycemic load compared to other staples of the Mediterranean diet, and so they should be eaten sparingly. And there are much better sources for resistant starch, such as oats and beans, which have more resistant starch than a potato and a much lower glycemic load.

The Extras

You won't find french fries or mashed potatoes on the Mediterranean diet, but potatoes do show up in soups, roasted with other vegetables, or in combination with diverse ingredients, such as in a classic French Salade Niçoise (page 182) or a Spanish Tortilla (page 209). But consider what *else* is in that Niçoise salad: green beans, olives, some fish, a hard-boiled egg, tomatoes, onions, and capers, all dressed with an olive-oil vinaigrette. Potatoes are only a part of it, not the main event. This is a theme you'll see over and over again with so many food preparations on the Mediterranean diet. There are foods that we erroneously tend to put front and center (meat and grains come to mind), but that Europeans wisely use as a small part of a larger whole meal—and therefore they don't overeat that particular food.

The Ligurian coast of Italy is famous for a dish that would seem to be a plateful of contradictions: pasta with potatoes! But consider how it's prepared. The pasta is tossed with pesto made with extra-virgin olive oil,

basil, pine nuts, garlic, and parmesan cheese. In addition to some sliced boiled potatoes, the dish traditionally features generous amounts of blanched fresh green beans—and you won't be served a super-sized portion. The ingredients and their proportions are what make it Mediterranean.

SWEETS

The Basics

When someone is wrestling with whether or not to have dessert, or wants an afternoon cookie or two (or a dozen), I advise the person to ask him- or herself this question: *What are you celebrating?*

Dessert with fruit or dark chocolate is part of the daily Mediterranean diet, but sugar- or honey-loaded treats are enjoyed only from time to time. On occasion, it's fine to have a sweet treat or a dessert, but choose carefully. Don't celebrate with junk. A perfect chocolate mousse that is absolutely scrumptious might be worth it if the moment is special. But cookie-dough ice cream on a regular old Tuesday night? It's not worth the price your body (and blood sugar) will pay. Besides the treat itself, always consider the occasion. Are you having a slice of cake because it's your birthday, or is it just another office party? (And is it a great cake, or is it stale and hardly worth eating?)

Whether or not you're trying to lose weight, eating sugary treats is a sure-fire way to damage your health.

The Extras

If you've been to Italy in the summer, you've seen it: hordes of people, including skinny

Italians (and other Europeans), indulging in gorgeous ice cream cones that resemble works of art, in every color of the rainbow. But . . . *they are on holiday.* It's *their* special occasion, and gelato is a summertime treat, not a staple of the Mediterranean diet. (Go back to that same town on a February evening and you won't see the same parade of people polishing off their stracciatella, the Italian take on chocolate chip.) And you'll find parallel situations in every Mediterranean country. Desserts are for celebrating, not snacking.

If you do have a craving for something a bit lighter than gelato—and it is a special occasion—Mediterranean countries have perfected icy concoctions such as the Italian granita and the French sorbet, made from frozen fruits, fruit juices, and purées—with no cream. However, they are still exceedingly sugary! Treat, treat, treat.

And finally, if you're thinking that the real problem with desserts is the sugar and that you can get around that by using artificial sweeteners, note that many chemical sweeteners kill off billions of healthy gut bacteria—for more on this, see Chapter 6 on gut health. If you must have sweetness, choose something flavored with honey—local and organic—it is better than anything flavored with chemicals.

We've now worked our way through every major food group—all the way up to the minor ones—and it's time to put all this knowledge to work, and learn about the active, social lifestyle that supports this diet so well.

One of the most effective uses of a low-glycemic Mediterranean diet is for weight loss and maintenance. And based on the results I've seen among my own patients over the years, I can assure you that the Mediterranean Method works. If your goal is to be trimmer and stay fit for life, you'll want to learn about my "skinny twist" on this traditional diet in the next chapter.

3

THE
MEDITERRANEAN
METHOD
FOR
WEIGHT
LOSS

If you want to lose weight—and especially if you've tried numerous diets or plans without success or lasting results—there is no better way than a Mediterranean style of eating, especially my Mediterranean Method.

It's more effective than a low-fat diet plan, and because the food is so appealing, it's considerably easier to follow than more restrictive diets such as low-carb, Paleo, or Keto plans. Even better, you won't just shed pounds and lose inches; you'll also enhance numerous aspects of your health, from lowering your risk of heart disease to improving your gut health and protecting your brain. Those multiple benefits, borne out by extensive research, are why the Mediterranean diet consistently outranks other eating plans as the best overall diet on the planet.

A few years ago, Dr. Joseph G. Mancini and his colleagues evaluated five randomized weight-loss trials involving more than 1,000 patients on different weight-loss regimens (low-fat, low-carb, etc.) who were followed for over 12 months. This 12-months-plus follow-up time is especially impressive because it means that researchers were able to track whether or not a diet delivered long-term weight-loss results—the true marker of success.

Unfortunately, we're often swayed by headlines and hype from short-term studies of trendy diets that show weight loss over 6 to 12 weeks, but generally all that weight (plus another 5 pounds or so) comes back. What is more deceiving are the weight-loss books touting, "Lose up to 10 pounds in 10 days." The reality is that you can only lose at most 1 to 2 pounds of fat per week. Any additional weight you lose means you are losing water, or far worse, you are losing muscle mass.

The Mediterranean eating plan, according to the meta-analysis of patient data in the Mancini study, was equally effective for weight loss as a low-carb eating plan (such as Paleo), and more effective than a standard low-fat eating plan. Here's another plus: when low-fat and low-carb diets are compared, followers of a Mediterranean diet showed more improvement in lipid and metabolic profile measures, including better cholesterol levels, blood sugar, and blood pressure. The average long-term weight loss among Mediterranean diet followers ranged from 10 to 22 pounds—and the weight stayed off throughout the 12-month follow-up period.

Even for those with Type 2 diabetes, the Mediterranean diet turns out to be the best path for weight loss. In a different meta-analysis of nine randomized dietary trials with over 1,000 patients, researchers concluded that when a Mediterranean diet was compared to the American Diabetic Association diet, a low-fat diet, or a low-carb diet, once again the Mediterranean diet showed superior results for blood sugar control, weight loss, and lipid profile changes.

To me, the idea that you could lose 10 to 22 pounds (and keep the weight off), improve your blood sugar and cholesterol profiles, and lower systemic inflammation, all while enjoying delicious Mediterranean food, sounds almost too good to be true. But . . . it *is* true. Still, research is one thing; real life—including your personal goals and challenges—is another. You can adapt the Mediterranean diet for long-term, sustainable weight loss through everyday eating when you use my Mediterranean Method—my "skinny twist" on this traditional eating plan.

But first, let's see what we can learn about weight control from one particular Mediterranean population who famously eats (and drinks) quite well yet stays trim and healthy: the French.

French Women (and Men) Really *Don't* Get Fat—and Here's Why

THE BESTSELLING BOOK *French Women Don't Get Fat* by Mireille Guiliano is as much about attitude as it is about what to eat (and not just for women). How do the French, who have a reputation for drinking wine, eating cheese, and enjoying bread, stay thin and live longer than most Americans and those in the rest of the Western world?

Researchers named this phenomenon "the French Paradox" in the 1980s, when

they observed that the French consumed dietary cholesterol and saturated fat from dairy products and meat, yet had low rates of heart disease. Meanwhile, British and American populations with the same cholesterol and saturated fat intake had much higher rates of heart attack and stroke. And to make it even more of a paradox, as mentioned, the French who ate this way were considerably thinner.

The lessons we can learn from France about weight control are similar to those offered by Spain, Italy, and other regions along the Mediterranean Sea, where there is far less obesity than what we experience in the United States. Consider that the obesity rate in France is just under 10 percent, while in this country it is more than 35 percent—that is, we have 300 percent more people who are overweight.

As a physician, nutritionist, and clinical researcher, I've been studying the French paradox for decades—but I've also had personal experience living in France, working and cooking on a sailboat cruising along its Mediterranean coast, as well as visiting my wife's French relatives and sharing many a home-cooked meal with them. Here's what I've learned about how they stay slim while still indulging in three of their most famous "food groups." If you read between the lines, you'll see a few themes emerging, including moderation, the quality of the food itself, and an active, less-stressful lifestyle.

WINE

Initially, researchers were quick to attribute the French health paradox to red wine consumption (see box on facing page) and likely, some of the health benefits of moderate red wine consumption do play a role—but as you'll see it's only a partial role.

The reality is that the French drink less wine now (and less alcohol overall) than they did in past decades, and wine consumption per capita has dropped—though it's still considerably higher than American consumption.

The French drink about 52 liters (about 54 quarts) of wine per person per year, compared to 12 liters (about 13 quarts) in the United States. Or, to put that into bottles, the French drink roughly 70 bottles of wine (much of it red) each year, and the Americans drink about 16 bottles. (However, we consume far more beer, and more hard liquor, too.)

That is an average of 1 serving of wine per person per day, certainly consistent with healthy living. France consistently produces more wine than any other country on earth (with Italy sometimes taking the lead, depending on annual harvests). Still, how is it that the French drink more wine—and all the calories that go with it—yet don't have as much heart disease or get the equivalent of American beer bellies?

We know there are health benefits to consuming 1 to 2 servings of red wine per day, as the pigments in red wine block oxidation and lower inflammation (see pages 38–39). But here's something more important that may unravel the paradox when it comes to weight control: In France (and other Mediterranean countries), *wine is consumed with food, and the food that is served is simply healthier than what is on the average American dinner plate*, in part because it's so much higher in fiber, especially from plant foods such as vegetables, fruits, beans, and nuts—all featured on the Mediterranean diet.

Wine also has a very low glycemic load. A glass of red wine has a glycemic load of zero, while an 8-ounce serving of lager beer has a glycemic load of 7.5, and a 12-ounce beer is 12.7. That means that beer has more than 500 percent more sugar load than wine.

When you consider that many people might drink 3 to 6 beers per day, that sugar load is huge, helping explain the term "beer belly."

The French eat nearly *twice as much fiber* as Americans, consuming on average a bit over 20 grams per day. Not only does fiber contribute to a healthy heart, but it also makes

Is It Just the Wine?

Some researchers have attributed the lower rates of cardiovascular disease among the French to red wine in particular. One theory surrounding the French paradox is that red wine makes blood platelets less "sticky," and therefore less likely to clump up and ultimately promote an arterial blockage. Another idea is that resveratrol, a compound with known anti-inflammatory and antioxidant properties found in the skin of red grapes (and therefore, red wine), is the reason for all those healthier French hearts. However, the dosage of resveratrol in 1 to 2 servings of red wine is fairly small—fifty times less than you could achieve with resveratrol in a supplement form. To reach supplement dosages (200–250 mg of trans-resveratrol per day), you'd have to drink copious amounts of red wine—but those benefits would be totally canceled out by the excessive amount of alcohol required. The reality is that there are many biochemically active compounds in red wine, not just resveratrol; and all these compounds combined produce anti-inflammatory and other benefits.

you feel fuller and more satisfied at mealtime. You won't overeat, and you won't be starving between meals.

The real secret to staying thin is probably on the plate, not in the glass.

CHEESE

In France, cheese-making is practically an art, and the variety of cheese you'll encounter there is staggering. It would be quite difficult *not* to eat cheese if you lived in France! But, like other Mediterranean dwellers, they consume high-quality cheese in modest portions, 1 to 2 ounces, traditionally enjoyed after a balanced meal served with red wine. A selection of cheeses might appear on the table with nuts and some sliced fruit, instead of a high-fat dessert that wouldn't sit well after a filling meal.

The cheese they eat is also rich in probiotics. In particular, Rochefort, camembert, and reblochon are loaded with healthy gut-supporting bacteria. In contrast, the cheese consumed in the United States is largely pasteurized and has far less flavor. French cheese is often raw, unpasteurized, and full of gut-friendly good bacteria and fungi to boost and balance our gut microbiome. There is ample data that a healthy gut microbiome helps you lose weight and keep it off, and that obesity is associated with bad gut microbes. (For more information on good gut bacteria and weight loss, see pages 111–114.) The French also enjoy plenty of gut-supportive yogurt and many other fermented foods.

Eating cheese doesn't make you skinny—but eating probiotic-rich cheeses and other fermented dairy as part of a Mediterranean diet will. (For more on probiotic-rich dairy, see Chapter 2.)

BREAD

What about all that bread? Like wine and cheese, bread in France is treated like a national treasure. But it's vastly different from the plastic-wrapped, mass-produced bread that fills our American supermarkets. For starters, the French have resisted the GMO (genetically modified organism) grain movement and still produce wheat from ancient strains that have not been tampered with. Non-GMO wheat produces less inflammation, and less inflammation is strongly associated with weight control. And we've already discussed the role of bread and bakeries in the Mediterranean (see pages 51–52), and the attitude toward eating bread: no mindless munching of a bottomless bread basket. A slice from a baguette is likely one-third the weight of a slice of bread we would eat with a sandwich. When the French do eat bread, they have a small portion and then stop; a baguette has a super-high glycemic load, however, so I'm not going to encourage you to start eating baguettes.

As for other grains, the French eat whole grains and in modest proportions, once again with a variety of vegetables and beans, flavored with fresh herbs and olive oil.

Vive la Différence—Better Food, Better Living

BEYOND WINE, CHEESE, and bread, the French tend to eat higher-quality food than we do—and they consume less of it, in part because what they do choose to eat is just more satisfying.

Part of this difference has to do with affordability and accessibility. In France and other Mediterranean countries, it's much easier for the average person to buy and bring home healthier food, and that's not just because of the plethora of open-air markets and the ingrained farm-to-table tradition. Even the produce and animal products sold in large supermarkets are generally produced with far fewer hormones, chemicals, and pesticides than their American equivalents. It's not that all European food is 100 percent organic—it isn't—but much of their meat and dairy is pasture-raised, and shoppers needn't spend vast sums or go out of their way to find it.

What does food quality have to do with weight loss?

First, chemical food additives such as artificial flavorings or colors, as well as pesticides and hormones, including growth hormones given to animals, can work in your body to make it harder for you to lose weight. (There is even a name for some of these weight-promoting toxins: obesogens, as in obesity.) Remember that if a factory-farmed chicken or cow ingests chemicals to make it bigger and fatter, and you eat that protein, you are ingesting the weight-gain-promoting chemicals as well. We are what we eat.

In addition, food quality can impact quantity, as in how much of it you'll consume. You might think, "But if it tastes that good, I'm going to eat a lot more!" (That's not a bad thing if we're talking about plant foods, incidentally.) Yet, if you do as the French do, and as the Italians, the Spaniards, and so on, you'll discover that you're incredibly satisfied with a 3.5- to 5-ounce portion of pasture-raised, perfectly seasoned and cooked steak, as opposed to eating a so-so slab of grain-fed, feedlot-raised steak that's twice or three times that size. A small serving of rich cheese is all you'll need—or want—and the same goes for other rich foods. In France, less really *is* more. But back home, if we can't break the habit of super-sized American portions, we'll continue to super-size our bodies.

Finally, there are a few lifestyle factors that are associated with maintaining a healthy weight. Food may be the game changer when it comes to weight loss, but being physically active is essential, especially for weight maintenance. The French were notoriously slow to embrace "le workout," and large, American-style stand-alone gyms and exercise studios have taken a while to catch on, even in big cities. Still, just a few minutes of people watching will bear out the fact that adults (and children) are fitter and slimmer across

the pond, even without Crossfit or Soul Cycle. That's because they build physical activity into their daily routines, primarily through more walking. When they do exercise, they don't emphasize the "work" in "workout," as most activities are things like leisurely games of tennis, tending a garden, cycling, playing soccer, or going for a swim.

On the other hand, we tend to have an all-or-nothing attitude when it comes to exercise, especially when using it for weight loss (never effective on its own, but potent if you combine it with a change in your food). "If I don't run five miles a day, five days a week, then there's no point!" The American can-do attitude can be a gift in some situations, but not in this case.

A better strategy is to make incremental, doable changes to boost your physical activity levels: an extra walk every day, taking the stairs, parking farther away to increase your steps, turning your walk into a walk-run, and so on. And if you do desire a structured exercise routine, find one that fits your lifestyle. Don't join a gym if it's located in a part of town you never go to, especially during rush hour. Instead, sign up at the one that's a block from your office—and that has classes (and showers) available before or after work, or even during lunch. (And never join a gym if you loathe gyms—you are setting yourself up for failure.) Be practical, and you're more likely to follow through on your commitment.

The more relaxed French attitude toward exercise—don't make a big deal out of being active, just do something you *like*—is a reflection of one other lifestyle factor associated with a healthy weight: Like other Mediterranean dwellers, the French are less stressed, overall, than average Americans. When it comes to food, they enjoy long, unhurried meals, often with family to whom they have closer connections, or with friends, a ritual that goes hand in hand with their *joie de vivre*. Sharing a meal with dear ones is a lot better for your heart—physically and emotionally—than a fast-food dinner for one, eaten in front of a screen.

High levels of unmanaged stress, we know, stimulate the hormone cortisol, which makes you gain fat around your waistline and lose muscle mass. Not only do the hormonal effects of chronic stress make you gain weight but they also produce cravings and lead you to make bad choices when you are stressed out. My experience from having lived and worked in France is that the French do more to proactively manage their stress, and they have lower rates of obesity, plus less depression and anxiety as a result.

This isn't to say that we can't manage our stress—as you'll see, we can. But far too often our American approach to work and the business of daily life means that stress manages us. We'd be healthier and happier (and probably thinner) if we adopted Mediterranean traditions that naturally manage stress.

A Skinny Twist on the Mediterranean Diet

FOLLOWING A MEDITERRANEAN diet to maintain good health, including a healthy weight, is straightforward. Using it for weight loss requires a little tweaking, but you're going to love the results, and because of the food, you'll find it so much easier to stick with this "diet" than other weight-loss plans.

The Spain-based PREDIMED study, originally published in 2013, is the largest study to assess the long-term impact of the Mediterranean diet on cardiovascular health, and it involved over 7,000 people. At the same time, PREDIMED researchers collected data on weight loss among a particular subgroup of Spaniards—those living in the Canary Islands, who have the highest obesity rates in the country—comparable to those found in the United States. Though study participants had excellent outcomes with regard to other markers of cardiovascular health, their weight dropped modestly—only about 2 pounds. The Mancini study, however, cited at the beginning of this chapter, showed greater weight loss (10–22 pounds).

Because the weight-loss benefits on a traditional Mediterranean diet seem to be mixed, my Mediterranean Method uses an approach that I know for a fact to be quite effective: *a low-glycemic-load Mediterranean eating plan,* like the one I created for patients at my clinic.

You already know from Chapter 2 that the higher the glycemic load of a food, the greater an impact it will have on blood sugar levels. In addition to numerous health benefits, my patients who follow a combination of a low-glycemic diet and a Mediterranean diet—essentially what you're learning about in *The Mediterranean Method*—have achieved even better weight-loss results than what I've seen published in clinical trials using a traditional Mediterranean diet. In my version, the primary difference is that I *de-emphasize foods—such as grains—that can trigger spikes in blood sugar, insulin sensitivity, and cravings.*

Not only have my patients gained control over their blood sugar as they've lost weight—often 10 or 20 or 40 pounds and even up to 100 pounds—they have also improved their blood pressure numbers and cholesterol profiles, reversed arterial plaque growth, lowered inflammation, and increased their brain processing speed! (We'll discuss the positive cognitive benefits of the Mediterranean diet in Chapter 5.)

To lose weight with the Mediterranean Method, you don't count calories or grams of fat. You do, however, pay closer attention to portion size, especially for foods that have a high glycemic load. In Chapter 2, I outlined foundational foods to eat every day, foods to have several times a week, and foods that should be consumed occasionally. You can follow that same template, but in addition to watching serving sizes a little more closely, you'll want to reduce or even eliminate foods such as grains that have a higher glycemic load.

Here's what a "skinny Mediterranean" pyramid based on my method looks like:

A FEW TIMES PER MONTH
red meat,
limit desserts and potatoes

SEVERAL TIMES (3–5) PER WEEK
fish and seafood, poultry, eggs,
whole grains (limit portion size),
probiotic-rich dairy (including cheese)

DAILY
vegetables, fruits, beans, nuts,
olive oil and other smart fats, herbs and spices,
yogurt, dark chocolate, red wine, coffee, tea, water

FOUNDATION
outdoor activity and exercise, market shopping, group cooking,
relaxation, leisurely dining with social interaction, and mindful eating

The biggest difference with a low-glycemic Mediterranean diet involves cutting back on whole grains and flour products, including bread. Review the information on grains and cereals in Chapter 2 (see pages 47–48) and you'll see that white pasta, rice, and corn are high-glycemic-load foods; whole grains, including oatmeal, farro, bulgur wheat, and both whole-grain pasta and protein-enriched pasta are medium. (See the more comprehensive glycemic load table of foods in Chapter 8, beginning on page 154.)

If you were simply maintaining your current weight using the Mediterranean diet and you were very active, then having a 1-cup serving of whole grains (including whole-grain pasta) several times a week would be fine. But if your goal is weight loss, then *reduce the portion by half and cut back on frequency.*

A ½ cup serving of whole grains a few times a week may not seem like much, but you'll enjoy it as a small appetizer or part of your meal. And I don't mean you'll eat ½ cup of plain brown rice. Instead, try ½ cup of a whole grain like farro, mixed with ½ to 1 cup of vegetables, such as bite-sized cubes of roasted butternut squash and red onion, plus toasted walnuts, olive oil, sage, and a little goat cheese—or mix and match the herbs and vegetables of your choice, and add some grilled fish or chicken on the side to turn it into a whole meal. Combining grains with vegetables, olive oil, herbs, and spices is a satisfying way to eat whole grains, and it adds more flavor as well.

When you follow a Mediterranean diet, you naturally eliminate processed foods. If you haven't done so yet, cutting them out of your diet takes health-wrecking and weight-promoting excess sugar and trans fats

A Sweet Surprise You Won't Want: Hidden Sugars

Sugar has dozens of names. When you pick up a product and read the label, don't just look for the s-word—look for its many aliases. Here are some of the more common disguises for plain old added sugar: any kind of syrup (corn, malt, barley—all grain sources); cane products, such as cane juice (and of course "organic" cane sugar—it's still sugar even if it's organic); cornstarch; dextrose, fructose, fruit juice, glucose, high-fructose corn syrup, maltose, potato starch, sucrose.

Artificial non-caloric sweeteners such as aspartame, sucralose, and saccharine may appeal to those trying to cut calories for weight loss, but the reality is that they may cause as much harm and weight gain as sugar-loaded sodas, triggering cravings and disrupting your gut microbiome (see page 116). Even if you aren't trying to lose weight, there are absolutely no health benefits to be gained from consuming artificial chemical sweeteners. If you want to lose weight and you're a diet-soda drinker, you'll do better giving it up and opting for a serving of unsweetened iced tea or red wine with dinner. There are a couple natural sweeteners available, such as stevia, xylitol, and erythritol, and although for the moment they appear harmless, there is likely no weight-loss benefit to using them.

out of your diet altogether—and by sugar I mean corn syrup, "organic cane sugar," sucrose, and more (see the box at left for more sugar aliases).

To really boost your weight-loss progress, take it one step further and don't just go after sugary-tasting foods—*target foods that turn to sugar.* At the top of the list? Flour products—including bread and crackers. The idea isn't to never eat these foods again. Instead, it's to view them the same way you would view sweets and desserts—as treats to eat in small portions, every once in a while, not weekly staples that are part of a daily routine. (See pages 51–52 for more on how they can send your blood sugar on a roller-coaster ride.)

If you want pasta, have it as you do whole grains—in small appetizer portions or as part of a larger meal, and mixed with plenty of healthy ingredients. (As noted previously, you can now also find pasta with added chickpea flour; it tastes great, and it also has more protein and fiber, and less refined carbs than most pastas.)

Another trick with pasta is to cook it until al dente (still a bit firm), and then immediately remove it from the hot water. Overcooked pasta causes a higher jump in blood sugar levels than al dente pasta.

And of course, as you know by now, the more active you are, the more you can have. If you are physically active for 6 or more hours a day, like a farmer tending steeply planted vineyards or a fisherman pulling the day's catch from the Mediterranean, then you need extra calories, and you can tolerate the higher glycemic load from foods like whole-grain bread and pasta. If your work days are more like mine have been during most of my career—you work full time and overtime, your work doesn't generally involve breaking a sweat, and you are limited to going to the gym for an hour per day—then you're struggling to be more physically active.

If weight loss is what you want, reduce your intake of grains, including flour products and whole grains.

Why the Mediterranean Method Works for Weight Loss

THERE ARE MANY overall health benefits to be gained from following my low-glycemic take on the Mediterranean diet, but to flip the switch and turn it into an effective weight-loss strategy, I recommend you make the additional adjustments I've outlined in this chapter. If you're wondering why you'll finally get the results you've been searching for, here are the key reasons:

1. BECAUSE YOU EAT MORE FIBER

The Mediterranean diet is loaded with fiber, which makes you feel full and satisfied, meaning that you won't be hungry in two hours. Fiber absorbs water, expands in your stomach and intestines, and makes you feel satisfied. Fiber also slows the rise of your blood sugar after a meal, which decreases insulin production. That also contributes to curbing your hunger. And if you aren't craving foods between meals, chances are you'll eat less and you'll make better choices to help you lose weight.

Data from the National Weight Control Registry, a database that includes thousands of American adults who have lost at least 10 percent of their body weight and kept it off for at least one year, shows that one of the best food predictors of "successful" weight loss is fiber intake. Perhaps the second best predictor of long-term weight loss is vegetable intake. According to data from the registry, eating plentiful amounts of fiber-packed vegetables is associated with losing weight—and not gaining it back.

2. BECAUSE YOU CUT SUGARS

The second principle of the low-glycemic Mediterranean Method that yields weight loss is avoiding sugar, refined carbs, and processed foods. You know they impair your blood sugar control, cause insulin resistance—the

body's inability to respond to insulin, the hormone that regulates blood sugar levels—and worsen your blood pressure and cholesterol profiles; but did you know that eating foods like chips, donuts, pretzels, candy, and fried fatty foods (be they salty or sweet) will stimulate hunger and cravings? The food industry has designed certain snack foods to make you hungrier for more so that you'll keep eating and buying more—and as a result you'll gain more weight.

If you think that all you need is willpower to overcome cravings for certain foods—specifically those that turn to sugar in your body—please think again. Willpower is no match for hormonal drives that stimulate hunger, as the body has multiple hormones that regular hunger, satiety, and appetite. Sure, you can power through sometimes, but your food cravings are going to win in the end. But there is a way to defeat them: through balancing your blood sugar with low-glycemic-load foods—including those on the Mediterranean diet.

3. BECAUSE YOU EAT CLEAN PROTEIN

As mentioned, too many of the animal products—meat and dairy—produced in the United States are injected or fed chemicals and hormones to help them gain weight, grow fat, produce more milk, and earn a greater profit when they're taken to market—after all, ranchers sell beef by the pound. Once they're turned into protein foods for us, we ingest those fat-growing obesogens that are stored in the animal's flesh and fat—substances designed to promote weight gain. Eating "dirty" protein is a bad idea for any person—and a particularly bad idea for a person who wants to lose weight.

Besides hormones, feedlot animals are given antibiotics, but not for treating infection. Studies have shown that if we feed antibiotics to animals (or to people as well), those drugs kill off good bacteria and promote bad gut bacteria that stimulate weight gain and make an animal fat. That's good for profits but bad for people, because when we consume antibiotics, the same things happen—we gain weight, and the inappropriate use of antibiotics promotes drug-resistant bacterial strains that can make us very sick. (And remember that eating clean shouldn't be limited to animal protein; as discussed, pesticides and other "obesogens" used on food crops can also promote weight gain.)

4. BECAUSE YOU EAT THE RIGHT FOODS AT THE RIGHT TIME

When you eat your carbs and protein also impacts weight gain and weight loss. Eating plain yogurt or eggs for breakfast provides protein, and *protein in the morning* revs your metabolism (your calorie-burning capacity) and helps you burn fat. Protein also suppresses hunger and will help you get from meal to meal without reaching for extra food. If you eat breakfast, *aim to get close to 20 grams of protein* for maximal weight-loss effect.

The worst time to eat your carbs is first thing in the morning. Your cortisol levels are peaking in the early hours to wake you up. If you eat refined carbs at the same time your cortisol is already on the rise, your blood sugar will jump and you'll set off a metabolic roller-coaster ride. Yet, this is what happens when we eat American-style pancakes with syrup, fried hash browns, bagels and toast, pastries, donuts, breakfast cereals (refined flour), and juice.

Here's an idea you can experiment with that's popular in Mediterranean countries—partial intermittent fasting. Stop eating by 9 p.m. and don't eat again until noon—basically a 15-hour fast. Doing this a few days a week will mix up your metabolism in a good way, improve your insulin sensitivity, and help you avoid cravings during the day. You can have black coffee or tea (no sugar or milk).

If you're a breakfast eater, make sure you get protein, some fiber to promote a sense of fullness, and some hydration to keep you full and satisfied (water, coffee, tea—but not fruit juice).

Eggs are definitely back on the menu—enjoy your eggs in an omelet, frittata, or sunny side up. Besides eggs, you might be wondering what to eat for breakfast (try my recipe for Greek yogurt with berries and nuts). Before your mind flashes on an image of a classic European café with coffee and pastry galore, keep in mind that pastries aren't part of the Mediterranean plan—unless you're in Paris on vacation! I think your priority should be to get 20 grams of protein with some fiber, as mentioned.

Although not part of the traditional Mediterranean diet, one simple way to acquire the protein in the morning is through a protein shake made with high-quality whey or pea protein powder, fresh or frozen berries, and something green (spinach or kale), and a liquid like almond milk—fast, nutritious, and easy. (You'll find my basic recipe on page 168.) I have one shake a few times per week, even when I'm sailing on the Mediterranean!

5. BECAUSE YOU'RE MOVING YOUR BODY MORE

Only 18 percent of people who diet to lose weight increase their level of exercise to help them reach their goals. Yet, activity levels are a critical predictor of losing weight and keeping it off. There are many good reasons for being active, from keeping your heart healthy to lowering your risk for depression and boosting your brainpower. But here's one stand-out reason if you're trying to lose weight: upping your level of activity will get you to the finish line more quickly, and help you sustain your weight loss over the long run.

Any decrease in calorie intake (which you'll do without thinking if you stick to my low-glycemic Mediterranean plan) can trigger a drop in your basal metabolic rate, or BMR, which equals the amount of calories you burn at rest. On a diet, your body senses that you're taking in less energy (calories consumed), so therefore it adjusts your metabolism so that you expend less energy (calories burned) when you are sitting at your desk job or otherwise "at rest." However, when you combine eating fewer calories with doing more physical activity, you'll rev up your metabolism, including your BMR, and keep a robust calorie burn rate going all day—especially if you do activities that build muscle mass.

Aerobic activity that gets your heart pumping helps to burn calories, boost BMR, and increase your exercise capacity. Strength training is what builds muscle. Both are important, but note that muscle mass is what really turbocharges your BMR. Add 1 pound of muscle and you burn an extra 40 calories a day (even while you're sitting at your desk). Maintain that extra pound of muscle mass over one year, and that means you'll burn an extra 14,600 calories (given that you must expend 3,500 calories to lose 1 pound, that's about 4.2 pounds of weight loss)—which is terrific. If you think in terms of volume of fat, adding 1 pound of muscle would help you burn away about one football of extra fat!

The triple-threat approach—aerobic activity, strength training, and my skinny twist on Mediterranean diet—works. That's why some of my patients have lost not just 10 or 20 or 40 pounds but even up to 100 pounds, and through regular exercise and watching what they eat, they've kept it off.

6. BECAUSE YOU'RE ADOPTING A MEDITERRANEAN MINDSET

It's tough to make good choices when you're stressed out (and it's especially tough if those choices revolve around food), you're hungry, and you're trying to lose weight. When we're stressed, our hormones go a bit haywire. Cortisol spikes, as does ghrelin, the "hunger hormone"; if we're also sleep deprived (thanks to stress), we have a dip in levels of leptin, the hormone that helps us feel full and satisfied. Stress creates a perfect storm of cravings for certain high-fat, high-sugar foods that call out to our reptile brain—that primitive part of our cerebellum that controls things we don't think about, like breathing and body temperature. We want comfort foods like chips, cookies, cheeseburgers, french fries, ice cream, and alcohol . . . fat and sugar. And if we're not prepared with handy, healthy food choices, we succumb.

But if we're not stressed—if we're more social, more active, and more rested—we make better choices. Eating in a leisurely Mediterranean way with others is pleasurable and relaxing—and a stress buster. So is having fun, or meditating, socializing, or doing any number of activities that de-stress the brain and body. The Mediterranean mindset is synonymous with a relaxed, it-will-all-work-out attitude. Many Americans who travel to Mediterranean regions where midday traditions of a long lunch (and maybe a nap) are still observed grow frustrated, particularly if they are still trying to follow an American timetable. *The car rental is closed! The stores are shuttered! The person at the front desk is gone! Where is everyone?* Well, they're out enjoying lunch from 1 to 3 or 2 to 4 p.m. (and sometimes from 1 to 4) and they'll return in the late afternoon and work until 7 or 8 or 9 p.m., refreshed and relaxed after a nice lunch break.

If you're ever in a residential neighborhood of a small Mediterranean town at around 1 p.m., and few locals are on the street, listen closely. If windows are open, you'll hear the same noises, over and over—the animated hum of conversation, the clatter of plates, forks, and knives, plus the clink of glasses, some laughter—and that's the sound of low stress.

We'd do best to do as they do and *slow down*, and schedule some time for fun and relaxation, so take your time when it comes to eating. Put real food on a real plate. Sit down with others. And enjoy. Mediterranean people still work plenty of hours, although they typically end up with less screen time in the evenings than we do. But that's a small price to pay for serving good food and making mealtime a sacred and cherished ritual.

If you lived like this, you'd probably eat better, lose weight, and live longer.

How to Convert Weight-Loss Failure into Success: Janet's Mediterranean Method Story

JANET CAME TO SEE ME AT MY CLINIC BE-cause she wanted to lose weight and keep it off. She was 52, not yet menopausal, her two children were grown and had moved away, and she wanted her figure back.

She had tried diet after diet—low-fat, low-carb, and most recently, a ketogenic diet—and with each of these, she had lost 10 to 20 pounds over six to twelve weeks, and gained it back, plus sometimes an extra 5 to 10 pounds.

She was now 40 pounds above her normal weight. None of her favorite clothes fit. She didn't like how she looked in the mirror. Not only had she lost her libido, but her husband didn't seem to want sex anymore.

During my assessment, I learned that her primary physician had recently encouraged her to eat more whole grains and less fat, and do more aerobic exercise—and told her to use more willpower. As a good patient, she had whole-grain cereal with nonfat milk for breakfast, spent 30 minutes jogging on a treadmill machine five days per week, ate a whole wheat wrap with vegetables and chicken for lunch and drank a diet soda, and she had a packaged dinner heated in the microwave with some form of protein, a whole grain, and a token vegetable, plus no-fat, sugar-free ice cream for dessert.

Not only was she eating the wrong foods, but she was eating them mindlessly as well—breakfast and dinner in front of the television, and lunch while working at her computer.

She said she had cravings and wanted to eat sweets, chips, and ice cream all the time. Most days of the week she avoided those foods, but sometimes she would just lose control and binge. Despite all her efforts, she was still gain-ing weight. She was crying when she finished her story. Fortunately from her history, I felt confident that I could help her.

On exam and with further testing, it was determined that not only was she overweight but her muscle mass was low as well, impacting her ability to burn calories. Her basal metabolic rate—her ability to burn calories at rest—was very low, in fact half of what it should have been. She had high blood sugar levels, and high hs-CRP levels (a marker for systemic inflammation).

At the end of her assessment I promised her that I could help. She wouldn't lose a lot of weight in the first 10 to 14 days, but she would keep losing weight and wouldn't gain it back.

I had her start my Mediterranean Method eating plan. She loved the food. She had either an omelet in the morning or plain yogurt with berries, or she skipped breakfast. Lunch was a salad with extra vegetables, a vinaigrette dressing, and a clean source of protein, plus unsweetened iced tea (no more diet soda). She had nuts for an afternoon snack. Dinner was any of the amazing recipes listed in this book with one glass of red wine, and dessert was a piece of dark chocolate with a piece of fresh fruit. She wasn't to eat anything after 9 p.m., and two to three days per week she wouldn't eat the next morning and would fast until noon.

She continued to exercise five days per week, but two days were focused on strength training, she added interval training for her aerobic session one or two days per week, and did a yoga session on the weekend. She also took a walk with her husband either before or after dinner.

No more meals or snacks in front of the TV or computer—she had to eat with someone and talk about the food she was eating. She added two social outings per week, with friends or family, and aimed for seven to eight hours of sleep every night.

I put her on a supplement plan, making sure she took a good-quality multivitamin and met her needs for fiber, vitamins D and K, magnesium, and long-chain omega-3 fats. I also gave her a special probiotic capsule daily to support her gut microbiome.

Thirty days later, she had lost 7 pounds and both her blood sugar and hs-CRP levels were back to normal. At three months, she had lost a total of 18 pounds and her calorie-burning capacity was normal. She was very happy to say that her libido had improved, and so had her sex life.

By one year, she had lost 30 pounds and was happy and felt great. I was proud of her, and we looked for ways to fine-tune and continue her improvements over time.

When I reflect back, helping her attain her goals was fairly easy, as she was following standard medical advice. Before we met, however, she had been doing many things wrong. She needed to avoid processed food (such as the microwave dinners) and focus on Mediterranean diet staples—vegetables, fruits, beans, and nuts, plus clean protein with olive oil and herbs for flavor. She needed to meet her key nutrient needs and support her gut. She needed strength training to build her muscle mass. And she needed to manage her stress, add social interaction to her life, and use mindful eating with her meals.

Janet was amazed by her results and how easy the program was to follow. Because it's such a realistic plan, you could achieve similar results.

Mediterranean Your Way: For Weight Loss

IF YOU'RE LOOKING for a precise calorie count for weight loss, that's not part of my Mediterranean Method. Everyone's goals are different, but assuming you're looking for weight loss without stress—whether it's 5 pounds or 50 or more—the "rules" I've outlined so far are clear, and you can put them to good use as soon as you're ready to prepare your next meal. Here they are:

- **Choose low-glycemic foods**—this is essential. (See chart, page 154.)

- **Reduce portions,** especially with regard to whole grains.

- **Consider eliminating all flour products.** If you do this, you'll break the cycle of cravings and overeating.

- **Eat at least 30 grams of fiber a day,** mainly from vegetables, fruits, beans, and nuts.

- **Aim for 20 grams of protein at breakfast.** A protein shake is a simple solution.

- **Experiment with intermittent fasting** (see page 149) to rev up your metabolism 2–3 days per week.

- **Use your body:** If you already exercise, do a bit more; if you don't, start. Use a combination of aerobic and strength-training exercise for maximum effects.

- **Be mindful:** Slow down and enjoy your food and the life you have—and banish stress (see page 146).

4

THE MEDITERRANEAN METHOD FOR HEART HEALTH

Cardiovascular disease (CVD) impacts 93 million adults, nearly 37 percent of the U.S. population, at a cost of $330 billion yearly. It kills more people than all forms of cancer combined. Many women think of breast cancer as the primary cause of death among females, yet for every one death caused by breast cancer, six women die from heart disease. Dying from heart disease is tragic—but from my perspective, surviving a heart attack or stroke but being left utterly debilitated is worse.

I know all too well the impact CVD can have, not just on the individual but also on the people around them. A heart attack could leave you with advanced heart failure, dependent upon oxygen to survive, unable to use the toilet without being too short of breath to require help. A stroke could leave you unable to walk, care for yourself, or speak. I've observed these grim outcomes of CVD firsthand as a physician. Unfortunately, I've also seen this devastation up close in my own family, as both my mother-in-law, Joy, and my stepfather, Chuck, suffered from heart disease and ended up disabled by its many complications; and my dad, Arpad, died of heart failure at age 95. Those experiences have motivated me, through my work as a physician, writer, and speaker, to help others protect their heart health—I never want you or your loved ones to suffer from cardiovascular disease.

Fortunately, heart disease is highly preventable. We can stop 90 percent of all CVD events with the right lifestyle changes. (Combined with proper medical treatment and healthy living, we could probably wipe out the additional 10 percent as well.) One of the best ways to halt CVD before it takes hold is through diet—specifically, moving away from the nutrient-poor Standard American Diet with its high payload of refined carbs, bad fats, and toxic additives from processed foods, and replacing it with a Mediterranean diet.

We Know the Mediterranean Diet Is the Solution

IT'S NOT JUST wishful thinking that you can eat well, live well with a less stressful Mediterranean approach to life, and avoid CVD. For the last seventy years, researchers have been documenting evidence that a Mediterranean eating plan and lifestyle can reverse and prevent heart disease.

In the mid-1950s, an American physiologist and public health expert named Ancel Keys—known for having developed K-rations for World War II troops—became a vocal advocate for the Mediterranean diet. Keys had spent extensive time living and working in Italy, and had studied the almost nonexistent rates of heart disease in the southern regions, where inhabitants adhered to a traditional Mediterranean diet. Eventually, he would create his Seven Countries Study, which compared data on diets and rates of CVD in the United States, countries in southern Europe versus northern Europe, Japan, Canada, and Australia. Though in later years that work would be used controversially (to hype low-fat diets as the only solution to heart disease, while blaming fats and ignoring the role of sugars in CVD), Keys can be credited with putting the heart-protective benefits of the Mediterranean diet on the map.

Much later, another study came along that would have a major impact on my career. In 1994, French researchers published the Lyon Diet Heart Study. Participants, all of whom had experienced a previous CVD event (heart attack), followed either a Mediterranean diet with added healthy fats or were placed in a control group that followed what was thought to be a prudent low-fat diet. After four years, the researchers compared the Mediterranean diet group to the control group, and noted that those following a Mediterranean eating plan had much lower rates of recurrence of CVD, including heart attacks and strokes. Switching to a Mediterranean diet, researchers concluded, was as or more effective than taking statin medications in reducing cardiovascular events. If the Seven Countries Study got people thinking about the heart-healthy potential of the Mediterranean diet, it was the Lyon Diet Heart Study that firmly confirmed its value in preventing heart disease.

The Lyon Diet Heart Study findings confirmed for me that diet and lifestyle changes were essential to guarding against CVD, and could be used in addition to (even instead of) medications or surgery. Granted, it is easier for a physician to prescribe a drug like a statin than to change a person's dietary habits, yet patient willingness to follow a Mediterranean eating plan has been fairly high, and it comes with no drug side effects.

Statins—the go-to drug for lowering LDL "bad" cholesterol—for instance, are potential lifesavers when offered to the right patient, but one side effect is that they can raise blood sugar levels; another side effect is memory loss, plus they can cause muscle damage and pain, a drop in testosterone levels, and liver inflammation. Studies have shown that statins reduce rates of heart attack in high-risk men, but adopting a Mediterranean diet not only lowers the incidence of heart attacks and strokes for men *and* women—appearing to be equally effective to statin therapy—but also helps with weight loss, lowers the rates of new cancers, and decreases overall death rates as well. (That said, *no one should stop a medication without their doctor's advice.*)

In 2003, reinforcing the findings from the Lyon Diet Heart Study, a large study in Greece, conducted by the Harvard School of Public Health and the University of Athens, showed that following a Mediterranean eating plan would reduce heart attacks and strokes. From 2011 to 2012, additional studies showed that even non-Mediterranean populations had less CVD events if they followed a Mediterranean diet.

And then, in 2013, the large-scale, landmark PREDIMED study with over 7,000 subjects, conducted in Spain and published in the *New England Journal of Medicine*, made headlines all over the world and affirmed the CVD-fighting reputation of the Mediterranean diet.

PREDIMED study participants were men and women between the ages of 55 and 80, all of whom were at high risk for CVD; they either had Type 2 diabetes or had at least three major CVD risk factors, including smoking, high blood pressure, poor

cholesterol profiles, overweight/obesity, or a family history of CVD. They were divided into three groups:

- The first group followed a Mediterranean diet, but each person was given 1 liter of extra-virgin olive oil to consume per week.

- The second group also followed the Mediterranean diet, but participants consumed at least 30 grams (1 ounce) of nuts per day.

In following the Mediterranean eating plan, both groups also increased their weekly servings of fish (by an extra 0.3 servings) and legumes (by an extra 0.4 servings per week.)

- The third group ate a low-fat Western diet, similar to the original low-fat American Heart Association diet.

For those in the first two groups, the results showed that by following a Mediterranean diet and adding the extra liter of olive oil or the nuts, *the rate for all cardiac events and strokes dropped by 30 percent*. The results were so dramatic that the study was stopped one year early, as it seemed unethical to leave people in the third group on the standard low-fat diet.

Not only has the PREDIMED study shown a reduction in CVD events, but additional published studies have demonstrated that a Mediterranean diet with additional healthy fats decreases the incidence of dementia, improves kidney function, lowers rates for Type 2 diabetes, reduces depression, improves bone density, and even reduces the risks from some forms of cancer. As for weight loss, all three groups lost weight, but the first two groups, who ate more healthy fats, lost more weight than those in the low-fat group.

The EPIC Greek Cohort study, published in 2012, and with nearly 24,000 participants, evaluated adherence to a Mediterranean eating plan for more than ten years in relation to cardiovascular events. Researchers also compared glycemic load with detailed dietary histories in all these patients. Those with the highest adherence to the Mediterranean diet and lowest glycemic load scores had the lowest rate of CVD events. And, if these individuals were overweight or obese, the benefits from following a Mediterranean diet combined with low glycemic load was even stronger. These results, as well as several other studies that support the EPIC findings, suggest that we can eliminate 40 percent of all heart disease prevalence, and 50 percent of the deaths associated with cardiovascular disease, by combining a Mediterranean diet with a low glycemic load.

Since 2013, additional studies continue to produce irrefutable evidence that the closer we follow a Mediterranean eating plan, the less heart disease there is. In addition, more recent research has shown that combining a low-glycemic-load eating plan with a Mediterranean diet is the most effective way to prevent cardiovascular disease events—precisely the Mediterranean Method I'm suggesting in this book.

If you've been looking for a scientifically proven, research-supported way to lower your risk of heart disease—without medications or surgical interventions, but with an easy-to-follow diet that you are sure to enjoy—you have your answer.

Why It Works

THE #1 CAUSE of heart disease isn't high cholesterol levels (despite what you might hear from statin drug commercials). The #1 cause is actually elevated blood sugar levels and eating too much sugar and refined carbs. When you control your blood sugar and get to the root cause of heart disease, other CVD risk factors will fall into line. The Mediterranean Method is the key to this kind of control. It also:

- Improves blood pressure control and helps reverse hypertension.

- Promotes weight loss and better weight control (see Chapter 2).

- Improves cholesterol profiles, because of the healthy use of smart fats from olive oil, nuts, and seafood, instead of excessive fats from red meat and fatty dairy.

- Lowers inflammation and oxidation, because of the diet's high polyphenol content (colorful plant pigments); lower inflammation and oxidation are strongly associated with a decrease in cardiovascular events.

UNCLOGGING YOUR ARTERIES

Cardiovascular disease is driven by the growth of arterial plaque—the fatty material that gets deposited along the lining of your arteries, mostly from eating unhealthy foods. The combination of elevated cholesterol levels, elevated blood sugar levels, and inflammation gradually form a lining of arterial plaque along your arteries. The worse you eat, the more plaque you form. The closer you follow a Mediterranean diet and lifestyle, though, the less plaque you will grow over time.

Many people think that heart attacks occur because this buildup of plaque eventually blocks blood flow through the arteries, like a drain pipe that narrows to a critical point due to an ever-increasing buildup of sludge. But the reality is that most heart attacks, strokes, and sudden cardiac deaths occur because a small arterial plaque thickening, perhaps blocking only 20 to 40 percent of the artery wall, pops like a pimple on your skin. In medical circles, we call the bursting of this lesion a *plaque rupture*. The plaque rupture releases chemicals into the blood, which can cause the artery to clot, immediately blocking blood flow. If this happens in an artery in your heart, we call that a *heart attack*; when it happens in an artery in your brain, we call that a *stroke*. Nearly 80 percent

or more of heart attacks and strokes occur because small, baby-sized plaques rupture, with an explosion of soft plaque into the arterial openings and subsequent clotting.

Here's what comes as a surprise to so many: This rupturing can occur most often years before your arterial plaque has time to calcify, thicken, and harden. If we want to prevent heart attacks, strokes, and sudden cardiac death, then we need to avoid arterial plaque formation and plaque rupture that triggers these devastating events. That's where the Mediterranean diet comes in.

Following a Mediterranean eating plan helps prevent plaque growth and plaque rupture in several different ways. First, it lowers blood sugar levels, blood pressure, and cholesterol levels—all important risk factors for arterial plaque growth. The Mediterranean eating plan also decreases inflammation, the typical cause for plaque rupture. And if you do have plaque rupture, a Mediterranean diet helps decrease clotting, thereby reducing your risk for a heart attack or stroke.

In a major analysis of six randomized clinical trials that compared a Mediterranean diet with a low-fat diet for reducing CVD risk factors, with a total of 2,650 participants, researchers concluded that the Mediterranean diet was superior not only for weight loss but also for lower blood pressure, better cholesterol profiles, and improved blood sugar, as well as lower inflammation. That is an encouraging outcome, but what impact can the Mediterranean Method have on the growth of arterial plaque?

Among patients at my own clinic who followed my low-glycemic version of a Mediterranean diet, not only did I see improvements in weight, body fat, and waistline, as well as better cholesterol, blood pressure, and blood sugar regulation, but I also observed the all-important shrinkage and reversal of arterial plaque growth—especially among my patients with advanced cardiovascular disease. As a preventive approach to targeting the plaque that leads to heart disease, the Mediterranean diet delivers.

ASSESSING YOUR RISK

There are a few tools your health-care provider can choose from to determine your risk of CVD, but one, in particular, stands out.

The first is *stress exercise treadmill testing.* This type of testing is looking for advanced cardiac artery blockage, as once your arteries are more than 70 percent blocked, that is when you start having angina (chest discomfort, fatigue, and/or shortness of breath) with activity (such as climbing stairs), and that is when your treadmill test becomes abnormal. I think this type of testing is terrific for measuring fitness, as well as blood pressure and heart rate response to exercise, but in terms of a way to measure arterial plaque growth, it is too late, only looking at end-stage disease. Many people will have had a heart attack, stroke, or have died from heart disease before their arteries became 70 percent blocked.

Another common test is the *cardiac CT.* A chest computed tomography (CT) scan will measure calcium in the arteries of your heart. The higher your calcium score, the more calcified plaque exists in your arteries, and that increases your risk for a future cardiovascular event. There are a couple of important limitations to cardiac CT scanning. The first is that any CT scan is a radiation exposure and thereby increases your lifetime risk for cancer (approximately a 0.3 percent increased risk of cancer for each scan you have). The second, probably more pressing concern is that CT scanning measures only old calcified plaque. It doesn't measure new, soft plaque that typically grows within a plaque lesion that has the potential to rupture. Soft plaque is the most dangerous plaque, and you'll want to know if you have it or not.

By far my favored method for measuring arterial plaque is ultrasound technology, or *carotid IMT,* which measures the *intimal media thickness* (IMT plaque growth) in the carotid artery—the big artery in your neck that conducts blood from your heart to your brain. With a noninvasive carotid IMT, plaque growth can be easily measured through the gentle placement of an ultrasound probe on the back of your neck. There's no radiation, no need for drawing blood, and it takes about 10 minutes, total.

Studies have shown that 95 percent of the time, the carotid arteries, the heart arteries, and even the arteries in your legs grow arterial plaque at the same rate. Therefore, if you measure the plaque thickness in the carotid artery, 95 percent of the time you'll get the same measure as if you measured other arteries, including to the heart. Even the Prevention Group of the American Heart Association considers carotid IMT testing to be an excellent way to assess future cardiovascular disease risk.

For the last fifteen years I have used carotid IMT testing in my clinic to determine whether a patient's arterial plaque is growing, shrinking, or staying the same. The average

American increases his or her arterial plaque at a rate of 1 to 1.5 percent per year. Yet patients who followed my low-glycemic-load version of a Mediterranean diet have experienced more than a 10 percent *decrease* in arterial plaque growth over five to ten years of follow-up.

Whether or not you know—from testing—your exact level of arterial plaque, you may have picked up this book because you are concerned about it. Data published from my clinic show that several factors can positively influence your ability to slow, halt, or even reverse plaque growth. Interestingly—though perhaps not surprisingly—these same factors, which I'll expand upon starting on page 85, are common features of following a Mediterranean diet and lifestyle:

- **FIBER INTAKE.** With its emphasis on vegetables, fruits, beans, and other plant foods, the Mediterranean diet is loaded with dietary fiber.

- **FISH INTAKE (food or a fish oil supplement).** The best food source for long-chain omega-3 fats is cold-water fatty seafood—and eating fish is part of this plan.

- **HEART-FRIENDLY NUTRIENTS (such as magnesium, vitamin K, potassium, and vitamin D).** Magnesium and vitamin K abound in Mediterranean foods, and spending time outdoors provides sunlight for making vitamin D.

- **FITNESS.** A Mediterranean lifestyle is an active lifestyle, where you learn to incorporate walking and other activities into your day, besides traditional workouts.

- **LOSING BODY FAT.** Multiple studies have shown that you lose weight and body fat by following a Mediterranean diet and lifestyle. (See Chapter 3.)

- **LOWER BLOOD SUGAR AND CHOLESTEROL LEVELS.** As the research shows, following a Mediterranean diet and lifestyle improves blood sugar and cholesterol levels.

- **DECREASE IN INFLAMMATION.** Many components of the Mediterranean diet reduce inflammation levels. (See the box on page 86.)

- **STRESS REDUCTION.** Depression and anxiety rates are far lower in the Mediterranean region than in the United States, in no small part because a Mediterranean lifestyle means being connected to your community, including eating meals leisurely with family and friends.

YOU CAN CHANGE YOUR (ARTERIAL) AGE

How would you like to turn the clock back on your heart and make it ten years younger? That's essentially what happened to hundreds of my patients who reduced their arterial plaque thickness through my low-glycemic-load Mediterranean Method diet and adopting lifestyle changes in line with the factors above, such as being more active and lowering stress. As mentioned, most people who follow the Standard American Diet are adding arterial plaque at a rate of 1 to 1.5 percent per year. But my patients were moving in the opposite direction, shrinking plaque thickness by more than 10 percent—thereby shaving about ten years off the age of their arteries. (On average, it took 2.3 years for this magnitude of plaque regression to occur.) Not only did they halt and reverse plaque growth, but they also showed improvements in their weight, body fat, and waistline, and also improvements in their cholesterol, blood pressure, and blood pressure.

From Cardiologist Dr. Stephen Sinatra: "A dream come true"

Stephen Sinatra, MD, internationally recognized cardiologist, best-selling author (The Sinatra Solution: Metabolic Cardiology)*, and a personal friend and colleague, has been a long-standing advocate for the Mediterranean diet, even before it became highly popular. He and I discussed why he considers this eating plan to be "a dream come true." He knows that when patients follow it, they have improved blood sugar control and insulin sensitivity, decreased inflammation, lowered blood pressure, and improved cholesterol particle size and LDL/HDL ratios. He sees the dominant use of olive oil as a critical component of the benefit of this program, but cautions that olive oil should be certified by groups such as the COOC (California Olive Oil Council) as 100 percent olive oil, as many olive oils, including those sourced from Europe, are diluted with inferior oils, such as canola oil. He also recommends following many aspects of the Mediterranean lifestyle, in addition to the diet.*

Eating for a Healthy Heart

WHICH FOODS ON the Mediterranean diet lower your risk of heart disease?

The short answer is just about all of them do (and *red wine* to go with your meal may help as well). That said, it's the *colorful plant foods—vegetables, fruits, beans, nuts, extra-virgin olive oil, and herbs and spices*—that are the standouts. Besides providing most of the calories (and delicious flavors) in the Mediterranean diet, these foods are bursting with plant pigments (flavonoids and carotenoids) that lower inflammation and help prevent arterial plaque formation.

- **Beans** are worth special mention here because we don't eat them nearly as frequently as they do in most Mediterranean countries, where they show up at meals almost daily. Consuming beans improves your blood sugar and cholesterol profiles, lowers inflammation, and promotes powerful antioxidant activity—decreasing arterial plaque growth.

- **Extra-virgin olive oil,** the primary fat in the Mediterranean diet for cooking and dressings for salads and vegetables, is also worth emphasizing. It's a heart-healthy source of fat, in contrast to butter (even if it's organic) that at best might be considered a "neutral" fat—one without benefits.

- **Herbs and spices** are much more prevalent in the Mediterranean diet and in my method. They make food taste fantastic, but have the added benefit of blocking inflammation and taking the place of excessive and unhealthy amounts of added salt and sugar (which are overly prevalent in the Standard American Diet and damage our hearts).

- **Seafood** (at least 3–5 servings per week) has anti-inflammatory properties that block arterial plaque formation and lowers inflammation.

What to Avoid

BESIDES WHAT TO eat for a healthy heart, there are also *foods to reduce or avoid* altogether, as they do in the Mediterranean:

Let's start with *red meat*, which rarely takes center stage on Mediterranean menus. Instead, it is served only two to three times per month, or used in small portions for flavoring (pieces of meat in a soup or small bits of bacon with vegetables)—and it almost always comes from pastured, organically raised animals. When it comes to heart disease, the latest research shows some controversy as to whether saturated fat and red meat intake increases your risk for a heart attack or not. However, we do know that toxins (hormones, antibiotics, pesticides) in land animals that accumulate in the fat can block insulin sensitivity and deregulate blood sugar, potentially increasing the risk for heart disease.

By contrast, in the Mediterranean, people choose leaner sources of protein (and smaller servings). For instance, *poultry* portions are smaller there, typically 4 to 5 ounces served three or four times per week. This provides a clean and lean source of protein, without excessive saturated fat. *Eggs*, organic and cage-free, are eaten a few times a week as well—another source of lean protein.

What about *whole grains*? As previously discussed, the more active you are, the more you (and your heart) can tolerate—but most of us don't get enough exercise to justify the quantities of whole grains (not to mention white-flour products like pasta and bread) that we typically put on our plates. Whether it's whole-grain flour or white flour, if we're not getting enough activity, we can't handle the excess blood sugar load and the subsequent stimulus that promotes the growth of arterial plaque.

As for bad fats, a Mediterranean diet does not contain damaged fats that can promote inflammation, such as *corn or soybean oil* (or so-called vegetable oil blends). These mass-produced grain and seed oils are manufactured from pesticide-laden crops, and are processed at such high temperatures that they oxidize and become pro-inflammatory. And of course, a Mediterranean diet does not include the absolute worst fat: heart-toxic *hydrogenated (trans) fats* that are found in processed foods. I always tell patients that eating trans fats is like pouring embalming fluid into your body, as these fats ultimately cause your arteries to harden.

The consumption of sugars and refined carbs—dominant in *processed foods*—is the #1 predictor for a heart attack and stroke. Their absence in the Mediterranean diet goes a long way toward explaining low rates of heart disease.

Nutrients to Help Prevent Arterial Plaque Growth

AFTER PERFORMING THOUSANDS of arterial plaque measures and comparing those results with patients' detailed nutrient intakes, I have been able to identify minerals and vitamins that have helped predict plaque growth and regression. The most important heart-protective nutrients we found were:

- Fiber
- Long-chain omega-3 fats
- Magnesium
- Vitamin D
- Vitamin K
- Potassium

FIBER

Fiber intake is likely the most important deficiency among people who follow the Standard American Diet. If you were to make only one dietary change to improve your overall health, eating more fiber would probably yield the most benefits—and that includes benefits for your heart. And ideally, you would get your fiber from eating vegetables, fruits, beans, nuts, and seeds—staples of the Mediterranean diet. Assuming you get plenty of exercise, you could also include some fiber from unprocessed whole grains. Here's why

fiber protects your heart (and keeps you feeling great, in general):

- It suppresses appetite and cravings and helps you to feel full and satisfied, which helps weight control.
- It dampens the rise in your blood sugar and insulin levels after a meal.
- It decreases inflammation.
- It lowers blood pressure.
- It improves your cholesterol profile.
- It helps remove toxins from your system.
- It prevents constipation.
- It feeds the healthy bacteria in your gut (the microbiome).

Try to eat at least 30 grams of fiber every day. To keep the math simple, just pick ten servings of fiber daily. Many plant foods—like the examples that follow—average about 3 grams of fiber per serving:

- 1 cup of vegetables
- 1 cup of fruit
- ¼ cup of beans (½ cup of cooked beans makes a double fiber serving)
- 1 ounce (1 handful) of nuts
- 1 cup of cooked whole grain (oats, bulgur wheat, farro)

Here's one combination for hitting your target of 30 grams per day:

- 3 cups of vegetables (most vegetables have about 3 grams of fiber per cup)
  —*Broccoli, kale, green beans, tomato, fennel, chard, asparagus*

- 2 cups of fruit (most fruits have about 3 grams of fiber per cup)
  —*Best are berries for their lower glycemic load, but enjoy apples, oranges, figs, melon, and pears, too*

- ½ cup of beans (most beans have 15 grams of fiber per cup)
  —*Black beans, chickpeas, lentils, pinto beans, red beans, cannellini*

- 2 ounces of nuts and seeds (2 handfuls, most nuts have 3 grams of fiber per ounce)
  —*Almonds, hazelnuts, pistachios, walnuts, pecans, macadamias, flax seed, chia seed*

- 1 ounce of dark chocolate (1.5 grams of fiber)
  —*Must be 74 to 80 percent cacao to count as dark chocolate*

The Mediterranean Diet Shuts Down Inflammation

Extra-virgin olive oil, according to research, is able to turn off inflammation-producing genes in your body, thereby slowing the aging process and lowering your risk for heart disease. Italian herbs—garlic, rosemary, thyme, oregano, basil, and parsley—also have powerful inflammation-blocking properties. And when you add olive oil and herbs to seafood, a Mediterranean staple, you get a delicious meal that's an anti-inflammatory powerhouse.

Cold-water seafood, especially wild-caught salmon, gets all the headlines in this country for its long-chain omega-3 activity, but for those living along the Mediterranean Sea, sardines are perhaps the most popular food source for long-chain omega-3 fats. These tiny fish eat low on the food chain and have a fairly short life span, meaning that they accumulate far fewer PCBs, less mercury, and fewer toxins than even wild-caught salmon. They are loaded with healthy fish oil, and they also have an abundance of

Co-Q-10, an energy-producing compound needed by heart cells.

In Europe, fresh sardines are typically served grilled, drizzled with olive oil and lemon juice and flavored with garlic, as either an appetizer or a main course. However, it is hard to find good-quality fresh sardines in the United States, where typically they're canned and eaten during a meal or as a snack. To people who do not enjoy sardines, they may not appear nearly as appetizing, but they're still an excellent food choice—just be sure they come in BPA-free cans and are packed in a healthy oil, such as olive oil, rather than the commonly used cottonseed oil. See how I use sardines with a Spanish Mixed Salad on page 185.

Prolonged inflammation of your arteries causes high blood pressure and accelerates plaque growth. But the Mediterranean diet naturally lowers your levels of inflammation system-wide, including your cardiovascular system.

I've had patients tell me, "But I can't possibly eat this much fiber-packed food in one day! Five cups of vegetables and fruit? Plus beans?" My response is that a 30-gram list of fibrous foods like that here is nearly all the food you need in one day—and fiber should be a priority for heart health. Just add olive oil, herbs and spices, and some fish or clean protein, and a bit of red wine with dinner. Mix and match as you wish—and your meals will look very similar to what you'd find in the Mediterranean.

LONG-CHAIN OMEGA-3 FATS (COMMONLY CALLED OMEGA-3 FATS OR FISH OIL)

Long-chain omega-3 fats are good for many aspects of your health, especially your heart. They come from seafood, in particular cold-water fish, shellfish, and seaweed. Great sources are wild-caught salmon, sardines, anchovies, herring, sole, mussels, oysters, clams, and seaweed. (See pages 44–46 for a longer discussion of seafood sources of omega-3s.) Omega-3 fats:

- Reduce your risk for heart attack and stroke

- Decrease inflammation

- Prevent dangerous heart arrhythmias

- Lower abnormal triglyceride levels (a form of cholesterol)

- Prevent blood clots

- Improve cognitive function

- Reduce joint pain

Studies show that these benefits are stronger when omega-3s are consumed in food, rather than as fish-oil supplements.

If you're following a Mediterranean diet, you would ideally have fish and seafood three to five times per week, and you'll meet your omega-3 nutrient needs nicely.

If you are vegetarian, you can consume daily servings of seaweed (such as 1 cup of seaweed salad in a Japanese restaurant), or take a DHA extract from a seaweed supplement. For a vegetarian, a 500 mg daily dosage would be sufficient.

If you don't get enough omega-3s through dietary sources, I recommend a pill or liquid source that offers *1,000 mg of DHA and EPA daily.*

IF YOU ARE SUPPLEMENTING, CHOOSE WISELY

Unfortunately, there is a lot of "fishy" fish oil out there; but armed with some facts, you can make informed choices. Here's one tip for starters: Avoid buying mass-marketed fish oil from a big-box chain store or vitamin store or from an unvetted internet source that sells suspiciously cheap supplements. (See www .drmasley.com/resources for some trusted vendors.) Here are two points to keep in mind when supplementing:

1. DOSAGE ISSUES: You'll want to choose a supplement that offers 1,000 mg (combined) of DHA (docosahexaenoic acid) and EPA (eicosapentaenoic acid), the two most crucial long-chain omega-3s, combined with diluted omega-3 components.

The most recent research shows that DHA is better than EPA at improving lipid profiles, decreasing inflammation, and lowering triglycerides, all key for heart health. But many manufacturers offer supplements with higher levels of EPA (in part because it's cheaper than using more DHA, but also because of older research). For instance, you'll find that a typical 1,000 mg supplement contains about 500 mg EPA, 400 mg DHA, and 100 mg of other mixed omega-3 fats. Some forms even have 70 to 80 percent EPA and only 10 to 20 percent DHA; I suggest avoiding those EPA-enriched formulas. If you could find pure DHA, that would be ideal, but it's very expensive and difficult to locate a source. All things considered, including cost, a fish oil containing 600 mg EPA and 400 mg DHA is the most reasonable option—just not less DHA to EPA than that ratio.

2. CONTAMINATION CONCERNS: Here's the unfortunate truth about most fish oil sold in the United States: it is rancid and it tastes awful. That's because it was cheaply extracted, poorly processed, and improperly stored; and as a result, its molecular components have broken down. The majority of Mediterranean countries would ban most fish oil produced in the United States because it doesn't meet their quality standards. Good-quality fish oil should taste pleasantly fishy—like fresh wild salmon—and it shouldn't stink like a fish market stocked with yesterday's unsold catch.

You get what you pay for. If you can't supplement with high-quality fish oil, then don't take it.[*]

MAGNESIUM

My published research shows that adequate magnesium intake is one of the most powerful predictors for limiting arterial plaque growth and arterial plaque regression over time, based on initial and follow-up carotid IMT measurements. Among its many functions, magnesium helps you:

- Lower blood pressure
- Improve blood sugar control
- Prevent muscle cramps and improve muscle function
- Avert migraine headaches
- Avoid constipation
- Improve cognitive performance

Take a look at the first three benefits—it shouldn't be a surprise that getting adequate magnesium would be good for your heart (a muscle). The minimum recommended daily allowance (RDA) for magnesium is 400 mg per day, but more than 70 percent of Americans do not meet this minimal goal. *If you can't get to 400 mg through food, you should be adding a supplement.*

---

[*] One additional point: The ApoE4 gene, which occurs in about 20 percent of the population, increases the risk for heart disease and high cholesterol levels (as well as memory loss). In research trials on fish oil, if researchers don't control for the ApoE4 genotype (and identify and control for them from trials), and everyone is given only 500 mg of EPA and DHA, then the entire group may not show any benefit. The results will be skewed if studies don't control for ApoE4. We know that people with the ApoE4 gene need bigger dosages to benefit (probably closer to 2000 mg of EPA and DHA daily), but they also benefit more from supplementation than people without the ApoE4 gene.

Many of the foods listed in the chart at right are a natural fit on a standard Mediterranean diet. As part of my Mediterranean Method, I've enhanced this list with additional choices to ensure you boost your magnesium intake. You won't find oat bran on most Mediterranean breakfast tables, but you will find plenty of seeds, nuts, beans, and green leafy vegetables—all good food sources of this heart-boosting nutrient.

If you plan to add a supplement to reach 400 mg per day, be aware that an inexpensive, widely sold form, known as magnesium oxide, is not easily absorbable and can cause intestinal distress. I tell my patients to avoid it. *Magnesium citrate* is your better bet: most people tolerate it better, and it can have a laxative effect, which is good if you need it. The best absorbed and best tolerated would be a protein-bound form of magnesium, such as *magnesium glycinate* or *magnesium malate.* But be careful: If taken in excess, all forms of magnesium can cause diarrhea. For additional information on finding the best sources of magnesium, please visit www.drmasley.com/resources.

Food Sources of Magnesium	
FOOD AND PORTION SIZE	**MAGNESIUM (MG)**
Pumpkin and squash seed kernels, roasted, 1 oz.	151
Brazil nuts, 1 oz. (1 handful)	107
Halibut, cooked, 3 oz.	91
Quinoa, dry, ¼ cup	89
Spinach, frozen, ½ cup (or 3½ cups raw)	81
Almonds, 1 oz.	78
Spinach, cooked from fresh, ½ cup	78
Swiss chard	76
Buckwheat flour, ¼ cup	75
Cashews, dry-roasted, 1 oz.	74
Pine nuts, dried, 1 oz.	71
Mixed nuts, oil roasted, with peanuts, 1 oz.	67
White beans, canned, ½ cup	67
Pollock, walleye, cooked, 3 oz.	62
Black beans, cooked, ½ cup	60
Bulgur, dry, ¼ cup	57
Oat bran, raw, ¼ cup	55
Soybeans (edamame), cooked, ½ cup	54
Artichoke hearts, cooked, ½ cup	50
Peanuts, dry-roasted, 1 oz.	50
Lima beans, baby, cooked from frozen, ½ cup	50

VITAMIN D

Vitamin D is an essential nutrient that not only benefits your heart and blood pressure but also helps your bone density, boosts the immune function, and even helps prevent death from cancer.

The most natural way to get your requisite vitamin D is through sun exposure (the sun stimulates vitamin D production from cholesterol in your skin). Since Mediterranean dwellers have a lifestyle that involves walking daily—as well as sitting outside in the sun to eat and talk about life—they likely do a better job meeting their needs for vitamin D, particularly those people who live in southern Spain, Italy, and Greece, as well as North Africa, than we do in most parts of the United States. They're simply outside more than we are, and under famously sunny skies.

Depending upon how much the sun shines where you live, you're either able to make vitamin D year-round or perhaps only six months of the year. With one hour per day of sunlight exposure in shorts and a tank top and no sunscreen, people in the southern and southwestern states (south of Atlanta to Dallas, and west to Santa Barbara) make enough vitamin D to meet their needs year-round. In the northern United States (as well as northern Europe), people only make vitamin D from sun exposure six months of the year, from late spring, through summer and into early fall.

If you get at least one hour of sunshine a day in clothing that exposes most of your skin, you likely don't need a supplement, but given the risk of skin cancer, it's not a healthy method for getting vitamin D. The alternative is to take a supplement—which is what I recommend. Based on data collected at my clinic in Florida (the Sunshine State), for my patients to reach a normal level (greater than 30 ng/mL (nanograms/milliliter), and preferably close to an optimal vitamin D level (40–60 ng/mL), I concluded that my patients need to take 2,000 IU of vitamin D_3 daily. But again, this amount may be different for you depending on how much sun exposure you get. I recommend that you talk with your medical provider about your vitamin D level and that you ensure you get enough vitamin D to meet your needs.

VITAMIN K

You and your heart need vitamin K for clotting (so that you don't bleed to death) and to prevent calcification of your arteries. Without vitamin K, you can't get rid of the calcium in your arterial walls, and they become stiff and hard—calcified—leading to high blood pressure, atherosclerosis, and heart disease. (Vitamin K plays a big role in how your body utilizes calcium; you don't want it in your arteries, but without adequate amounts, your bones lose calcium.) Unfortunately, most Americans don't meet even the minimal intake guidelines for vitamin K.

Vitamin K exists in two forms—K_1 and K_2—but you need both. That said, people on certain anticoagulation drugs should speak to their doctor before supplementing with K_1 or K_2. The blood-thinning drug warfarin (Coumadin or other brand names), for instance, decreases vitamin K coagulation activity; taking extra vitamin K from food or supplements can block the medication's action and could cause life-threatening clot formation.

VITAMIN K$_1$: You can probably meet your needs for vitamin K$_1$ through food, particularly green leafy vegetables, which are a big part of the Mediterranean diet. You'll see in the chart that follows that the staple of American salads—iceberg lettuce—doesn't count as a leafy green! (It really has very little nutritional value, let alone vitamin K.) The minimum amount for proper clotting is around 100 mcg of vitamin K$_1$ per day (90 mcg for women, and 120 mcg for men), but your arterial function is much better with *at least 200 mcg of vitamin K$_1$ daily*. For optimum function, many experts suggest *500 to 1,000 mcg daily*.

VITAMIN K$_2$: Vitamin K$_2$ is the more potent form of vitamin K, and provides additional cardiovascular health benefits (as well as bone benefits). This is especially important for people who already have known heart disease.

In the famous Rotterdam Study, which tracked risk factors for 4,800 people followed over ten years, greater dietary vitamin K$_2$ intake was associated with a decreased risk for cardiovascular disease. Researchers compared people who got less than 21 mcg of vitamin K$_2$ per day; 21 to 32 mcg per day; or more than 32 mcg per day. Those with more than 32 mcg per day had 57 percent less risk for heart disease than those with less than 21 mcg per day. Other studies have shown that 200 mcg might be a more optimal dose for people with heart disease.

Supplements provide a convenient way to increase intake for both vitamin K$_1$ and K$_2$ (particularly the latter, as it's difficult to get K$_2$ from food). You can find vitamin K added to multivitamins, fish oil, and vitamin D supplements. Again, visit www.drmasley.com /resources for additional information on vitamin K supplementation.

Food Sources of Vitamin K$_1$	
FOOD AND PORTION SIZE	**K$_1$ (MCG)**
Kale, cooked, drained, 1 cup	1,062
Collards, cooked, drained, 1 cup	1,059
Spinach, cooked (or ~7 cups raw), 1 cup	889
Beets, cooked, 1 cup	697
Broccoli, cooked, 1 cup	220
Brussels sprouts, cooked, 1 cup	219
Onions, raw, 1 cup	207
Parsley, 10 sprigs	164
Cabbage, cooked (or ~3 cups raw), 1 cup	163
Asparagus, cooked, 1 cup	144
Lettuce, iceberg, ¼ head	3

POTASSIUM

While every cell in your body needs potassium to function, your arteries in particular need it to dilate and keep blood pressure well controlled. Extreme lows and highs in potassium levels can cause irregular heart rhythms which can lead to serious and even deadly consequences if the heart stops beating. Potassium levels can be low if you aren't getting adequate potassium in your diet, but levels can also be lowered by some medications (in particular, diuretics).

The general recommendation for potassium is *at least 4,000 mg daily*. As with other heart-healthy nutrients in this section, most people in the United States don't get nearly enough—on average only about half that amount—which impacts arterial function. That might explain our population's high levels of hypertension compared to rates among people in the Mediterranean. (Muscle cramps are also a consequence of poor potassium levels.)

As you can see from the following chart, the Mediterranean staples of beans, fruits, vegetables, yogurt, and seafood are good sources of potassium.

Food Sources of Potassium	
FOOD SOURCES	**POTASSIUM (MG)**
Beans, 1 cup cooked	1,000
Fish (salmon), 6-ounce serving	1,000
Dark green leaf veggies, spinach or kale, 1 cup cooked	840
Dark green leaf veggies, spinach, 1 cup raw	170
Baked potato, with skin, 1 medium potato	930
Sweet potato baked with skin, 1 medium potato	550
Dried apricots, ½ cup	750
Baked squash, acorn or butternut, 1 cup cooked	900
Yogurt, plain, nonfat, 1 cup	625
Avocado, ½ cup	550
Banana, 1 medium	420
Mushrooms, 1 cup sliced	420

If you are concerned about your potassium levels, work with your doctor to make sure you're getting adequate amounts from healthy foods and, if needed, you can take a prescribed medication as potassium therapy.

Stopping Heart Disease Before It Stopped Him:
Vito's Mediterranean Method Story

VITO CAME TO SEE ME AT MY CLINIC FOR A full evaluation, worried that at age 50 he was destined for a heart attack. Over the last decade, he had gained 40 pounds, lost his energy, and felt short of breath climbing stairs. His primary-care physician wanted to start him on three new medications, for his cholesterol, blood pressure, and blood sugar. Adding to his anxiety, a close friend had recently died of heart disease. He looked truly worried.

After completing his evaluation, I was alarmed as well. His arterial plaque score, based on his carotid IMT, made him fifteen years older than his actual age. His cholesterol, blood pressure, and blood sugar levels were all in the danger zone, and unless he made drastic changes, he would need to take the medications his primary-care doctor had recommended, and perhaps a fourth for erectile dysfunction. I wouldn't have been surprised if he had dropped dead from a heart attack in the next year—not just because of his lab results but also because of the lifestyle he led that was the root cause. A successful entrepreneur, he was constantly on the go and worked in a high-pressure business environment, spending little time on self-care. He had a poor diet, was not getting the nutrients he (and his heart) needed, got no exercise, and seemed highly stressed—slipping further each day into a rapid, risky downward health spiral.

Fortunately, not only was his name—Vito—Italian but he had the bravado and determination of a proud Italian, as well. I planned to tap into this desire to succeed with my pitch to transform his life.

I gave him a choice. Either we could slow, but not prevent, his demise through medications that would likely make him feel overall a bit worse, as he would decline over time and merely postpone what was coming. Or, he could follow my low-glycemic Mediterranean Method, enjoying satisfying and delicious Italian and Mediterranean flavors, and adding specific nutrients as needed. He could also incorporate physical activity into his routine and find ways to manage stress. Then we would assess his response.

I assured Vito that I'd helped thousands of people just like him and that if he followed this plan, I was highly confident he would feel dramatically better, not need the medications, prevent a heart attack, and restore his *joie de vivre*. Would he give it a try?

Vito became one of my most faithful patients of all time. He followed my eating, activity, and nutrient plan precisely, and within a month he felt dramatically better. He loved the Mediterranean recipes and meal ideas. Within six weeks, he had lost 15 pounds and his cholesterol, blood pressure, and blood sugar levels were all normal. (His wife now joked that his libido had improved too much.) At the end of one year, he had lost 45 pounds, looked trim and fit, felt fantastic, and all his labs and health markers looked optimal. His carotid IMT plaque score had dropped by 12 percent, a twelve-year drop in arterial age.

Ten years later, he has kept the weight off and remains healthy, still following my program carefully—and with pleasure as he enjoys the diet and lifestyle changes, and is thankful for the life-changing (and probably life-saving) results. Vito still looks and feels awesome. I am proud of how effectively he lowered his risk for heart disease, turned his health around, and become so much happier. And I am confident that you can achieve these same results, too.

Mediterranean Your Way: For Heart Health

THIS REALLY IS the best way to eat—and live—for a healthy heart. The documented low rates of CVD in the Mediterranean, as well as research conducted there and around the globe (including my own), offer overwhelming proof that this diet can work for anyone concerned about heart health—wherever home may be. Here's a roundup of the major points:

- Assess your risk: Talk to your health-care provider about measuring your levels of arterial plaque—don't wait until you have a CVD event.

- Get plenty of fiber from Mediterranean staples like vegetables, fruits, nuts, and beans and long-chain omega-3 fats from seafood—and supplement with additional heart-protective nutrients, where needed.

- If you need to get your weight under control, see Chapter 3.

- Go beyond food to reduce your risk—get active and reduce stress.

- Make sure you're getting the nutrients you need for heart health—easy to get through food if you adhere to the Mediterranean diet.

- Follow *The Mediterranean Method* to reduce your risk—and share this food with loved ones to protect their hearts, too!

5

THE MEDITERRANEAN METHOD FOR A BETTER BRAIN

Though you might not need statistics to confirm this, extensive polls tell us that memory loss—dementia—is the most dreaded of diseases, more so than cancer or heart disease. A person eventually disabled by memory loss—including Alzheimer's disease, which causes 70 percent of dementia cases—loses his or her independence and personality, a devastating transformation to witness. And sadly, that person—once a devoted parent, dear spouse, or faithful friend—becomes a burden on loved ones.

It's not just an emotional hardship; it's a financial one, as well. Medical expenses related to the care of someone with memory loss make it the most expensive disease in America today, more than heart disease or all cancers combined. And rates of memory loss, dementia, and Alzheimer's disease are increasing at epidemic proportions, predicted to double over the next twelve to fifteen years. In the United States, there are more than 6 million people living with diagnosed Alzheimer's disease, racking up a cumulative medical bill that exceeds $215 billion per year. Globally the projection is more staggering; from now through 2050, numbers will go from 36 million to 115 million with Alzheimer's, a 320 percent increase! Despite decades of research, there is no known cure on the horizon.

But there are a few corners of the world where memory loss is uncommon, even among the very elderly. Early on in *The Mediterranean Method*, we explored the robust health and low levels of chronic disease among people who live in the Blue Zones (see pages 19-21), including the Greek island of Ikaria. Elderly Ikarians have about 75 percent less dementia than their American counterparts, and they live well into their 80s and beyond without memory loss, whereas half of all Americans who live past age 85 show signs of Alzheimer's disease.

Researchers have found similarly low levels of dementia among long-lived Blue Zone dwellers from Okinawa to Sardinia to Costa Rica and Loma Linda. Despite that geographical spread, we know that there are overlapping food and lifestyle habits among all these populations—plant-based diets featuring some of the same foods such as seafood, leafy greens, nuts and beans, as well as active lifestyles and low stress levels. And among the people of Ikaria, as well as Sardinia, that diet and lifestyle is 100 percent Mediterranean.

You've just read how the Mediterranean diet can prevent and reverse arterial plaque growth and the heart disease it promotes. What does that have to do with this chapter on memory loss and brain health? The answer is, plenty—because as you'll see, *there is a direct association between arterial plaque growth and cognitive decline*, including memory loss. As I've shown from my own research, and as numerous studies have demonstrated, arterial plaque is a powerful predictor of brain decline. And here's another link in this chain: Diseases of the heart and brain often are rooted in poor blood sugar control, which in turn leads to insulin resistance, pre-diabetes, and Type 2 diabetes—conditions that can literally starve and kill off healthy brain cells.

If you put it all together, it's clear that there's a solution and a way to break this cycle of heart and brain disease. The #1 cause of memory loss is insulin resistance, pre-diabetes, and Type 2 diabetes, all of which contribute to heart disease—but we know these conditions are almost entirely preventable and reversible through a low-glycemic-load diet and some lifestyle changes. If we can protect our hearts, then we can protect our brains the same way—with a Mediterranean diet and a healthier lifestyle.

Understanding Memory Loss in Order to Prevent It

DECADES BEFORE A person develops significant memory loss, he or she suffers from gradually decreasing brain processing speed. Processing—which differs from memory, the ability to retain and recall information—refers to handling information and knowing what to do with it. A person with decreased processing abilities and intermittent memory issues may show signs of cognitive dysfunction that include:

- brain fog

- difficulty concentrating

- forgetting people's names

- having to reread a passage because the person forgets what he or she just read

- misplacing glasses, phones, and keys

- forgetting why he or she walked into a room

- leaving a meeting at work, then not remembering the assigned tasks

Nationwide, we're seeing an increase in these early symptoms of cognitive dysfunction in younger and younger people in their 40s and 50s, decades before such issues might surface. And this decreased brain processing speed impacts not just job performance but also overall potential and personal well-being.

By contrast, in my own clinic I've seen my average patient *improve* brain processing speed over time, and in a randomized clinical trial I'll discuss later in this chapter, we saw a 25 percent improvement in executive brain function skills within just ten weeks—enhancements that have been maintained now for years. In my clinic and within the larger trial, you won't be surprised to learn that one cornerstone of this progress was embracing a healthier way of eating—a low-glycemic Mediterranean diet.

The Blood Sugar–Brain Connection

DOCTORS CAN MAKE an Alzheimer's diagnosis by confirming the presence of an inflammatory protein, beta-amyloid, found in a patient's spinal fluid or the brain itself. It turns out that the same enzyme responsible for breaking down insulin also clears out this telltale protein. But when blood sugar levels go awry, so does that whole process—and the result is brain dysfunction and accumulation of beta-amyloid.

Dr. Melissa Schilling at New York University, who broke new ground with her theories, describes the link between Alzheimer's and insulin resistance this way: When insulin levels go too high (which can happen from eating diets loaded with refined carbs), the enzyme's activity is diverted to insulin removal, not to the removal of beta-amyloid. But if we regulate our diets and get blood sugar under control, things go back to normal and the enzyme can do both jobs once more, removing beta-amyloid from the brain and insulin from the blood. (Note: There is an ongoing debate as to whether or not beta-amyloid is the cause of Alzheimer's disease or an indirect marker of the disease process, but its presence is a confirmation of the disease.)

If we consume diets loaded with refined carbs, including the Standard American Diet, setting off increased insulin production and eventually causing insulin resistance, Schilling says, we won't be able to prevent excess beta-amyloid from forming in our brains. But she goes on to predict that by reversing insulin resistance, we will avoid at least 60 percent of Alzheimer's disease diagnoses. I think the Mediterranean diet and lifestyle could help boost that percentage even higher, especially if we combine those changes with new cognitive testing methods and early intervention.

The bottom line is that insulin resistance causes memory loss. I believe that we can prevent and reverse insulin resistance and Type 2 diabetes 95+ percent of the time with a low-glycemic Mediterranean diet and other lifestyle changes, thereby helping to prevent dementia as well.

Nourishing the Brain: We Know What Works

AS MENTIONED IN the last chapter, the large-scale PREDIMED study famously measured the effectiveness of a Mediterranean diet, compared to the standard low-fat diet, in the prevention of heart disease. As part of the study, researchers also tracked the cognitive impact of these dietary interventions over 6.5 years on over 500 participants, all of whom were at high risk for heart disease. And the findings on bolstering brain health were as encouraging as the portions of the study that focused on reducing heart disease.

Participants were randomized to either a Mediterranean diet with extra nuts (1 ounce per day), a Mediterranean diet with extra olive oil (1 liter per week), or a low-fat diet (similar to the American Heart Association diet recommendations). In their data analyses, researchers controlled for multiple other variables, including age, gender, education, weight, smoking, family history of dementia, genotype, and many additional risk factors. All subjects had cognitive testing assessed after their respective dietary intervention.

Those in the two Mediterranean diet groups, whether they added extra nuts or more olive oil, had better overall cognitive scores compared to the low-fat group. After six and a half years, more participants in the low-fat diet group were diagnosed with dementia than those in the Mediterranean diet groups. Interestingly, the results also demonstrated that "dietary compliance" (the ability to follow the recommended eating plan) was higher with the Mediterranean diet than with the low-fat diet—confirming that it is easier to stick with it over the long term than to follow a standard low-fat diet.

The PREDIMED findings, as well as similar results from the EPIC study (see pages 77–78), are consistent with other research that set out to compare diet/lifestyle choices and cognitive function in a variety of populations. Despite the diverse participants—including Americans from different backgrounds—the resulting data consistently points to cognitive benefits from following a Mediterranean diet compared to following a low-fat eating plan:

- In France, the "Three-City" study focused in part on the consumption of olive oil and cognition in the elderly. In one subset of participants who were followed for five years, more than 1,400 adults over the age of 65 who adhered to an olive-oil–rich Mediterranean diet showed less cognitive decline over time.

- In New York City, the Washington Heights–Inwood Community Aging Project (WHICAP) has been tracking participants ages 65 and older since 1989 to study risk factors for Alzheimer's disease. WHICAP data also link greater adherence to a Mediterranean-style diet with a lower risk of developing mild cognitive impairment and with reduced risk of mild cognitive impairment conversion to Alzheimer's.

- Following a Mediterranean-style diet—including consumption of omega-3 fats

from fish—was also associated with slower rates of cognitive decline in the Chicago Health and Aging Project (CHAP), which has been tracking health and aging among more than 10,000 people on Chicago's South Side since 1993.

- Some researchers zeroed in on whether or not the Mediterranean diet could offer brain-protective benefits to Americans from different ethnic backgrounds, starting in their mid-40s—topics that had not been explored. In a group of more than 1,200 Puerto Rican adults, ages 45 to 75, greater adherence to a Mediterranean-style diet was associated with better cognitive performance and a lower risk of future cognitive impairment.

We know how the Mediterranean diet works to promote heart health through reducing arterial plaque formation, but how does it protect cognitive function? For one major clue, look to the diet's polyphenol-rich foods—including the nuts and olive oil that featured so prominently in the definitive PREDIMED study. These plant foods have anti-inflammatory and antioxidant properties. Inflammation and oxidative stress, which produce damaging free radicals, are closely linked to poor cognitive function and neurodegenerative diseases, including Alzheimer's. In other words, a Mediterranean diet seems to strengthen our antioxidant defense system and block inflammation as it enhances brain health. Specifically:

- B vitamins—folate, vitamins B_6 and B_{12}—are linked to better brain performance. Beans and legumes are a great dietary source.

- The antioxidants found in fruits and vegetables, as well as wine, coffee, and tea, are plant foods that pack a polyphenol punch.

- Monounsaturated fats—found in olives and nuts—are associated with improved cognitive function and lowered risk for cognitive decline.

After three years, participants in the PREDIMED study who followed the Mediterranean diet had increased levels of "total plasma antioxidant capacity" in their blood—meaning that they were better able to resist brain-damaging oxidative stress; those who adhered to the diet also had lower concentrations of inflammatory markers, including C-reactive protein, interleukin 6, and white blood cell counts.

However, not every study has shown that the Mediterranean eating plan protects against dementia. Study results with participants who were monitored after age 75, and followed for less than five years, have not been consistently positive. But as a reminder, the average age of participants at the onset of the PREDIMED trial was 67. It may be that the benefits of the Mediterranean diet are more protective if the diet is started at a younger age, and have a longer interval to yield benefits over time.

My recommendation would be this: the sooner you adopt the Mediterranean Method, the better off your brain will be! It's *never* too late to make positive lifestyle changes that will improve your health and longevity.

What Happens if We Go Beyond Food?

THERE'S NO QUESTION that the research comes down firmly on the side of the Mediterranean diet as a way to enhance cognitive function and slow or prevent progression to dementia—all by itself. Yet, what happens when you combine this heart- and brain-saving diet with physical exercise, mental exercise, and other lifestyle changes?

The FINGER study from Finland, conducted from 2009 to 2011, followed more than 2,600 subjects between the ages of 60 and 77 who had risk factors for heart disease and/or early signs of cognitive decline. Half the participants were randomized to a control group and were given general health advice, but were not asked to change their diets. The other half followed a Mediterranean diet, added regular exercise and cognitive training (puzzles and other tasks that challenged the brain), and received advice on how to reduce their risk for cardio-vascular disease.

Those in the control group, who received nothing beyond health advice, lost brain function and had greater progression to dementia. However, those in the multi-therapy intervention showed an improvement in cognitive function, and they had less cognitive decline.

Previously researchers had been concerned that asking study participants to make multiple changes at once would be overwhelming. What they discovered in the FINGER study was the opposite: The dropout rate was lower than expected and the compliance was greater than they'd hoped. Participants reported that they felt much better and were much more likely to stick with the multi-step intervention, more so than only doing one step at a time. (I also think they liked the food!)

At my own clinic, patients who combine dietary changes with other interventions (exercise, stress reduction, and more) for heart disease, Type 2 diabetes, and cognitive function are also likely to stay the course—because they love how they feel on so many levels. But it's not just about feeling sharper, stronger, or more fit—it's about what's actually happening to their bodies and brains.

I've done follow-up cognitive testing on patients for up to twelve years. We've also

---

Dr. David Perlmutter on Brain-Boosting Foods

Dr. David Perlmutter, a neurologist and the author of the popular and New York Times *bestselling book* Grain Brain, *and a long-time colleague and friend, tells me that he appreciates the brain-protective benefits of the Mediterranean diet, and in particular the nutrient-rich foods, the low amounts of refined carbs, the good fats, lots of seafood, the moderate dairy and minimal red meat consumption, and a bit of red wine.*

To improve upon it, he recommends adding more olive oil and more nuts—as was done in the PREDIMED study discussed earlier—and his other recommendations also echo my low-glycemic approach: limited portions of whole grains to keep the glycemic load low (though he feels the grain should be 100 percent gluten-free and fully unrefined). A diet like this, he says, would reduce the risk for dementia and other neurological diseases, as well as heart disease and cancer.

In recent years, Dr. Perlmutter has noticed a trend among some Mediterranean populations, as they've shifted to a less healthy, more fast-food (American) style of eating. I admit I've seen this too in my travels, particularly when I leave the smaller traditional towns along the coastal Mediterranean and head into the larger inland cities. "From a neurological perspective," he told me, "eating a Western pro-inflammatory diet will disengage frontal lobe brain activity and function, and engage the amygdala region of the brain (the fear center)." The result, he predicts, will be a population that is fearful, overly reactive and distracted, and far less focused, thoughtful, and calm.

Fortunately, from what I've observed, the Mediterranean lifestyle still has a powerful grip on many and is prevailing from generation to generation—in part because the lifestyle itself, beyond the food, is so satisfying.

shown that in a randomized trial using our recommendations for a low-glycemic-load Mediterranean diet, combined with activity and stress management over a ten-week intervention, that the average patient increases his or her brain processing speed and executive function by an amazing 25 percent. Meanwhile, the average American has a drop in brain processing speed over time.

To me, there is no doubt that the way to a better brain is through a better diet—combined with a healthier lifestyle—and it's Mediterranean in nature.

FIVE STEPS TO PROTECT YOUR BRAIN

From my clinical experience, I have discovered that combining the five interventions that follow—rather than relying on diet alone—offers a more effective, synergistic, and long-lasting strategy for improving brain function and preventing cognitive decline.

1. **EAT THE RIGHT FOODS.** Chockful of antioxidant and anti-inflammatory foods, the Mediterranean diet is an excellent starting point, but my Mediterranean Method is a low-glycemic version outlined in this book. Yes, all the Mediterranean diet nutrients are great for the brain, but since insulin resistance is the #1 cause for memory loss, doing more to prevent elevated blood sugar levels by ensuring you eat mostly foods with a low glycemic load is the best move. Chapter 2 walks you through the basics.

2. **ADD BRAIN-BUILDING NUTRIENTS.** You can get plenty of vitamins and minerals

from the Mediterranean diet, but as part of the Mediterranean Method, you'll want to boost your brain and mental sharpness with adequate amounts of these important nutrients highlighted—and for many people that may mean adding vitamin and mineral supplements.

Vitamin D. Several studies have found that low vitamin D levels are associated with a higher risk for cognitive decline and dementia, and people with higher D levels actually have larger brains compared to those with insufficient amounts. The active form of vitamin D stimulates the growth of brain cells. See page 90 for a full discussion on why you'll likely need to add a vitamin D supplement. Check with your health-care provider to check your level and to determine how much you need, but for most adults, *2,000 IU daily* is adequate.

Magnesium. Magnesium helps to shrink arterial plaque and improve blood sugar control, which ultimately will benefit your brain, as plaque formation is a risk factor for cognitive decline. It's also essential for proper messaging between brain cells. See the table on page 89 for some good food sources in the Mediterranean diet, including nuts, seeds, beans, and leafy greens. Aim for *400 mg daily*, first from food and then supplement if necessary.

Omega-3 fats. What helps the heart helps the brain—and omega-3 fatty acids, best obtained through cold-water fish like wild-caught salmon, sardines (a Mediterranean favorite), and herring, are invaluable. Long-chain omega-3 fats, or fish oil, protect your brain because they fight inflammation. When you select a fish oil supplement, note that some studies have shown that DHA is more effective than EPA in improving cognitive scores. See the discussion on pages 87–88 on how to ensure you get the right balance of DHA and EPA. For a longer explanation on seafood and omega-3s, see pages 44–46. *Eat seafood 3–5 times a week or choose to take a supplement with high-quality fish oil containing 1,000 mg of EPA and DHA daily.*

B vitamins (B$_{12}$ and mixed folates) and chromium—available from a good-quality multivitamin. Your brain needs B vitamins! Brain cells will actually die if they don't get enough vitamin B$_{12}$, which they use to convert glucose into energy. It's not uncommon to have permanent and irreversible nerve damage—and develop dementia—because of a B$_{12}$ deficiency. Mixed folates are a group of B$_9$ vitamins responsible for repairing cellular DNA and removing toxins. Folate deficiency is associated with depression, cognitive decline, and dementia, as well as heart disease. And chromium helps your body avoid insulin resistance—the most reversible cause of dementia. While you can get some B vitamins and mixed folates from beans and chromium from certain foods (including red meat, whole grains, and cereals—though I don't encourage their consumption because they will blunt the benefits of the Mediterranean diet)—the simple solution is to get all these brain essentials from a daily multivitamin, which is why I've grouped them together here. Pick a multivitamin with at least *100 mcg of B$_{12}$; 400 mcg of mixed folates; and 400–800 mcg of chromium.* For tips on choosing a quality multivitamin, see page 144.

Probiotic supplements. There is a documented link between a healthy gut—populated with beneficial bacteria—and a healthy brain, and building up the diversity of gut microbes is associated with reducing the risk of cognitive decline. While the Standard American Diet, along with overuse of antibiotics and substances like chemical sweeteners, can wipe out good bacteria, probiotic foods and supplements will restore the gut. (I'll focus more on this in the next chapter.) You can enjoy fermented dairy foods such as probiotic-rich cheeses, yogurt, kefir, and pickled vegetables and olives on the Mediterranean diet, and "feed" the good bacteria with fiber—at least 30 grams per day (see pages 85–87). But you want *billions* of microbes working for you. If you feel you're not meeting your needs through diet, and to really tune up your gut—and your brain—consider adding a supplement. Look for one with a variety of probiotic organisms, not just a few and a dosage of 25 billion or more daily. See pages 104–105 for more on choosing a probiotic supplement.

Other nutrients to consider are curcumin, MCT oil, and resveratrol.

Curcumin. Derived from the turmeric root and an essential part of Indian cuisine, this supplement has terrific anti-inflammatory properties. As it turns out, the cultures that consume curcumin (from turmeric in curries and other spice blends) have some of the lowest levels of dementia on the planet! You would have to all but abandon a Mediterranean diet and eat a *lot* of curry, however, to get its cognitive benefits, so look for a capsule form that delivers *500 mg of curcumin*. Note: You need high-quality "clean" curcumin easily absorbable by the body and uncontaminated by heavy metals, which is not always easy to locate. See the information on page 36 for more information.

MCT oil. Medium-chain-triglyceride oil is also associated with better brain function, though the studies to date suggest it's most effective in improving cognitive function in people who already have some memory loss, rather than as an outright preventive measure for healthy adults concerned about cognitive decline, but research is ongoing. MCTs break down into ketones, molecular by-products of fat-burning. In ketosis, which is generally achieved through fasting, the brain uses ketones for fuel, and for a variety of biochemical reasons, the brain responds well to ketones. In lab research, animals in ketosis had increased memory capacity and even brain growth. One option to boost ketone levels is to skip breakfast two or three days per week. But rather than fasting, you can get them from taking MCT oil, too. If you have some established cognitive issues, talk to your physician about starting a trial of MCT oil. It does have some gastrointestinal side effects, though they aren't serious for most people. If you are healthy and you want to test-drive the impact of MCT oil on your brain, take *10 grams to start and work up to 20 grams* over the course of about two weeks.

Resveratrol. This is the anti-inflammatory and antioxidant compound found in wine—particularly red wine (see pages 38–39). It helps with blood sugar control, which ultimately benefits the brain, but resveratrol also seems to boost blood brain flow and at least one small study shows that it has a positive impact on cognitive performance. Much of the research on resveratrol focuses on its role in preventing heart disease, but again, what's good for the heart is good for the brain. As mentioned earlier, however, you'd have to drink a lot of red wine to get the heart-brain benefits of resveratrol—too much, in fact, for your overall health. Instead, take *200–250 mg of trans-resveratrol in supplement form.*

3. EXERCISE YOUR BODY—AND YOUR BRAIN. As you probably already know, exercise is good for everything—from heart health to better sex—and you may not need extra convincing to make sure you make time for it. But just in case, consider the fact that exercise can help to reduce arterial plaque, as well as bring insulin sensitivity and blood sugar control back into optimal ranges—and all that translates into better brain health. Interestingly, aerobic activity (getting your heart pumping for 20 minutes or more) and strength training (stressing your muscles with weights or resistance bands) are independently important, and based on my findings you should do both.

In published data from my clinic, we showed that aerobic fitness was the most powerful predictor of improvements in cognitive function over time. My patients improved executive function up to 25 percent when they added aerobic exercise; executive function is the ability to process complex information and jump from project to project quickly. Strength training can be a great workout, and more muscle mass is the key to better blood sugar control. (The less muscle you have, the less capacity your body has to store glucose as usable energy after a meal; instead it ultimately gets stored as fat.) But strength training on its own is not associated with as much positive impact on cognition as aerobic activity has. The best way to exercise for brain health? Combine aerobic and strength training—and support your physical activities with a low-glycemic-load Mediterranean diet.

But don't stop with your body; work your brain, as well. Research tells us that the brain really is like a muscle: If you don't use it, it will shrink over time. But challenge it and it will grow, both functionally and in size. Cognitive activity (mental challenge and new learning) helps improve brain function and prevent memory loss. Besides crossword puzzles and Sudoku, maybe it's time to take up a musical instrument or finally learn that new language.

4. BE PROACTIVE ABOUT STRESS MANAGEMENT. Too much stress makes your head hurt—and it also hurts your brain. Acute stress is manageable—the deadline will pass, the scary movie will end, the traffic jam will break up. But chronic stress will cause chronic health problems, including cognition issues. Over time, unmanaged stress will keep your cortisol levels set to "high"—and blood sugar levels will stay elevated as well, increasing your risk for heart attack or brain-damaging stroke.

Take a lesson from the Mediterranean lifestyle, and don't wait until your stress levels are at a breaking point: It's not just good food—it's also a good life, featuring a more relaxed approach to daily living, with plenty of social connection and built-in ways to manage stress (like daily exercise in the form of walking). We'll talk more about that lifestyle in Chapter 8, but for now, note that ways to manage stress—through exercise, getting enough sleep, and taking up mindfulness practices like meditation, or maybe seeking outside help if you're dealing with a tough personal issue—aren't just ways to make you feel better; they are strategies for protecting your brain health and keeping dementia at bay.

5. GET TOXINS OUT OF YOUR LIFE (AND OUT OF YOUR BRAIN). We've already discussed the importance of choosing foods that are free of undesirable hormones, antibiotics, and pesticides; ingesting them will make you sick, and increasingly, research shows that environmental toxins—like BPA (see page 26)—can interfere with the body's ability to regulate insulin, leading to poor blood sugar control, which in turn damages brain function. Fortunately, when you choose a Mediterranean diet, you are also choosing unprocessed, whole foods that tend to be fresh, local, and frequently organic (including dairy and other animal protein), grown without pesticides and free of chemical additives. Still, there are a few "brain baddies" worth calling out:

Nitrosamines. Used in processed meats (such as deli meats and bacon), nitrosamines are associated with insulin resistance, neurodegenerative injury, and Alzheimer's disease. Mediterranean countries (and much of the rest of Europe) are generally more rigorous about banning chemicals and preservatives in their food supply, and you won't find nitrosamines in genuine cured meats such as high-quality prosciutto (the ingredients of this unprocessed meat are simply pork, salt, and time). Also, consider that European cured meats are considered a pricey delicacy, sliced paper-thin and served as an occasional appetizer. (In the United States, we think nothing of ordering a deli ham sandwich with a quarter-pound or more of meat!) As I don't expect our laws to change anytime soon, make sure that if you eat processed meats, such as bacon, choose high-quality products that are nitrosamine or nitrate free.

Mercury. We've known for decades that mercury damages the brain. Because of the oceanic food chain, it's what we call "big mouth" fish that tend to contain the most mercury: tuna, grouper, bass, kingfish, and swordfish. Stick to eating shellfish more often that is so prevalent and popular in the Mediterranean basin. You should be able to eat seafood two to five times per week if you stay away from big-mouth fish.

Inorganic copper. Our bodies need copper, but not the wrong kind, which is toxic. Organic copper in food—including Mediterranean staples like nuts, seeds, beans, mushrooms, and leafy greens—and in high-quality supplements is desirable. But a buildup of inorganic copper from sources like copper pipes and "copper salts" used in cheap supplements can be harmful. In fact, some experts have documented a link between Alzheimer's and inorganic copper, which has caused an increase in beta-amyloid production

in mice. Researcher and physician George Brewer compiled data that showed a correlation between inorganic copper content in public water supplies that use copper plumbing and the rise in Alzheimer's diagnoses.

Fortunately, even if you live with copper pipes (as many of us likely do), you can reduce your exposure to excess copper:

- Use a reverse-osmosis filter in the kitchen to remove inorganic copper from your home water supply, especially for drinking and cooking water.

- Don't use copper cookware.

- Choose supplements that are copper-free or that use only organic copper.

If you're looking for more detailed, practical strategies for protecting your brain, my previous book, *The Better Brain Solution*, offers an in-depth program for protecting and enhancing your cognitive function.

Fortunately, an incredible paradigm shift is occurring in the medical field today. Not that long ago, we didn't think there was much we could do to reverse memory loss and protect the brain from cognitive decline, including Alzheimer's disease. But we've learned, thanks to science, that it's just the opposite: By changing our diet and lifestyle, we can improve and heal our brains—well before advanced memory loss or a diagnosis of cognitive dysfunction—and the Mediterranean diet and lifestyle is a great way to begin.

A Better Lifestyle, A Better Brain: Claudia's Mediterranean Method Story

CLAUDIA WAS 49 WHEN SHE FIRST CAME TO see me, worried about early memory loss and having trouble focusing at work. An accountant at a busy firm, she was forgetting to follow up on tasks after meetings, and her boss had complained that she was making mistakes. Claudia's mom had developed Alzheimer's disease at an early age, and she wondered if she was experiencing early signs herself.

Things had been uneventful, healthwise, until about a year ago, when her divorce was finalized. As it turns out, Claudia's husband had done most of the food shopping and cooking. Now she didn't feel like preparing dinners just for herself. Her diet, she admitted, had gone downhill. She ate breakfast on the run, and lunch was usually a quick, rushed bite at her desk, in front of the computer. She was trying to follow a Paleo eating plan, but based on her description of typical meals and snacks, Claudia was relying on a lot of packaged foods and wasn't eating nearly enough vegetables, fruit, beans, or nuts.

On her evaluation, she was overweight (she had gained 18 pounds over the last year), her nutrient intake was poor, her blood sugar levels were elevated, and her cognitive function testing showed decreased brain processing speed. She certainly appeared to be at high risk for memory loss and to have early signs of decreasing cognitive function.

I asked her to try my low-glycemic Mediterranean eating plan, and to adopt some of the other lifestyle features as well, including a daily walk, eating more leisurely (no more lunches at her desk), enjoying dinner with a friend, and doing more socially. We agreed to repeat some of her testing after she followed the plan and reassess her status.

When she returned in six weeks, she said she was thinking much more clearly and felt more focused and productive, both at work and at home. Her boss had noticed an improvement in her job performance, and to her delight, she enjoyed shopping for fresh, appealing ingredients and cooking from the low-glycemic Mediterranean recipes I'd given her. She lost 10 pounds and her blood sugar levels were normal as well. Best of all, her brain processing speed had improved by a whopping 40 percent. She was thrilled and motivated to stick with our plan.

A year later she still felt terrific, her weight was back to normal, and her cognitive function remained very sharp. Like many of my patients, Claudia showed that you can improve your cognitive function with the right lifestyle changes. And given her family history, I believe that she had also stopped the cognitive decline that could have progressed over time to premature Alzheimer's disease.

Mediterranean Your Way: For Brain Health

- Understand the connection between heart health and brain health—and take steps to protect both, especially with diet and lifestyle changes like those in *The Mediterranean Method*.

- Don't rely on one intervention to save your brain. Combine a low-glycemic Mediterranean diet, exercise (both aerobic and strength training), stress reduction, supplementation, and toxin avoidance for a full range of benefits and protection.

- Focus on nutrients in Mediterranean staples that are especially brain boosting—like omega-3 fats from seafood and magnesium from beans, nuts, and seeds.

- Remember that there is no reason to wait until it's too late before you take steps to prevent and slow cognitive decline. Whether it's your own brain health or that of your spouse, a parent, or another loved one, who wouldn't want to have a better brain?

6

THE MEDITERRANEAN METHOD FOR A HEALTHY GUT

Even though we were taught that "germs" were nasty (and some truly are), our bodies are equipped with a sophisticated system of naturally occurring microbes—bacteria, fungi, viruses—that keep us healthy and protect us from illness and disease.

Collectively, this system is known as the microbiome, and it's composed of a staggering 100 trillion microbial cells that live on or in the human body—for instance, in the mouth, on the surface of the skin, and throughout the gastrointestinal (GI) tract. Our general immunity to illness is bolstered by maintaining a healthy, balanced microbiome, which is why we don't have to live in germ-free bubbles, why we can touch our computer keyboards and then rub our eyes without getting an infection, and why runny-nosed toddlers don't have to be quarantined.

More important, there is the specific intestinal or "gut" microbiome—those organisms that make themselves at home in the GI tract. Whether or not you follow trends in healthy living and wellness, you've undoubtedly heard a lot of talk about "gut health" and "good gut bacteria," as well as the gut microbiome.

There's a compelling reason why these gut-related topics are catching the attention of so many: It turns out that gut health—the balance and diversity of beneficial gut bacteria that make up the gut microbiome, as well as the integrity of the gut barrier that protects your GI tract—is closely related to overall health, not just that of the digestive system. A host of issues such as obesity, heart disease, and even brain disorders can be linked to the state of the gut microbiome.

Perhaps you're less concerned about the bigger microbiome/overall health picture and more interested in ways to address classic GI problems. These can range from commonplace complaints such as heartburn, gas, indigestion, or constipation to more complicated GI issues, including irritable bowel, gluten sensitivity, fatty liver disease, or leaky gut syndrome. Either way, whether it's mild digestive discomfort or a more serious bout of stomach troubles that are keeping you from regular activities, these issues great and small are stemming from what's going on in your gut. And not surprisingly, what we eat plays a critical role.

That may seem obvious, of course. Most of us don't have iron stomachs, and if we overindulge in a particular food or eat something rotten, our guts will send us a strong message, even as they send us to the bathroom or reaching for medication. Those moments are sharp reminders of what *not* to eat. But we've now learned, thanks to research on the gut microbiome, that there are many foods we should be eating to keep our guts in tiptop shape—filled with nutrients that boost the growth of beneficial bacteria—and some that we should reduce (or even eliminate).

You don't need to tack a list of these foods onto your refrigerator. All you need to do is follow *The Mediterranean Method* and you'll get a good gut feeling—and the good overall health that goes with it.

Gut Check: How It Works and What Can Go Wrong

TO BE MEDICALLY accurate, the "gut" isn't limited to your stomach and intestines. Instead, think of it as a twisting pathway that extends from your mouth, where food goes in, to the other orifice, where undigested food comes out the other end as waste. There's lots of action along the way—largely dependent upon the type of food that travels through this tubelike structure.

The GI tract (interchangeable here with the word "gut") has a huge absorptive surface area—about the size of a tennis court when spread out flat. For the gut to work properly, it must allow nutrients to be absorbed by the body, but simultaneously it must prevent food particles, toxins, and microbes from leaking into the bloodstream. This gatekeeping activity is the function of the "gut barrier" that lines the GI tract—a regulatory system that can allow or block certain substances from entering or exiting.

Beyond its filtering capacity, the GI tract needs to pass contents from one end to the other, produce digestive enzymes to break down food into tiny particles, and kill bad bacteria and microbes that threaten to cause infection.

In all these ways, the GI tract is both feeding and protecting the nutritional health of the entire body. When nutrient absorption is compromised, it doesn't just impact the GI tract but also impacts every organ in the body, including the heart and brain, as specific nutrient deficiencies can trigger many diseases. As examples, vitamin B_{12} deficiency can cause irreversible memory loss and nerve damage, and low calcium absorption can lead to loss in bone density and debilitating fractures.

Because the gut surface area is very large and is loaded with bacteria that must *not* pass into the bloodstream, the body's largest concentration of immune activity and microbe-fighting lymphoid tissue is in the gut. This means that GI problems are also the #1 cause of systemic inflammation, a major risk factor for heart disease, memory loss, accelerated aging, autoimmune diseases, and body-wide aches and pains.

The key to gut health depends upon two primary factors. The first is a healthy balance of gut microbes, commonly referred to as the gut microbiome. The second relates to the integrity of the GI lining or gut barrier, which should allow nutrients to be absorbed while preventing potentially harmful substances from escaping into the bloodstream. Let's look at how a healthy gut offers the body protection from disease, and what happens when the gut microbiome is disrupted.

Why the Gut Microbiome Matters

NEARLY 9,000 RESEARCH papers have been published over the last decade on clinical studies related specifically to the gut microbiome, and as we continue to establish links between overall health and gut health, it will likely remain one of the richest areas of research in medicine.

For the last 300 years, since the invention of the microscope, we have been aware of the existence of some of these microbes, but only very recently have we begun to discover their importance and impact on human health. Simply put, the right ones keep you feeling good and the bad ones can cause harm.

Beneficial microbes metabolize toxins and drugs, lower inflammation, help you absorb nutrients, and suppress appetite, which is why it's important to "feed" good gut bacteria and simultaneously control the growth of harmful microbes.

This just-right balance is key. Little more than a decade ago, investigators proposed that the gut microbiome might be contributing to obesity. Now many published studies show that by manipulating gut bacterial populations—and getting the right balance of microbes—you can convert thin mice into fat mice and fat mice into thin mice. Treatment protocols that revolve around achieving the right levels of certain microbes are now being developed to help people with obesity.

In recent years, the microbiome has been linked to many other health issues, especially neurological diseases. Autism, Parkinson's disease, dementia, and depression have been linked to abnormal gut bacterial populations—perhaps an overgrowth of undesirable microbes or a depletion of health-boosting ones. As with obesity, treatment protocols for these problems commonly include therapies to support the gut microbiome.

Even heart disease in now being associated with the gut microbiome. Gut bacteria impact many of the important risk factors for cardiovascular disease, including blood sugar and cholesterol levels, blood pressure control, and obesity.

Adopting a diet rich with nutrients that nourish friendly microbes and regulate overgrowth of problematic ones will help you improve your baseline health and lower your risk for an array of chronic conditions. The Mediterranean diet in general, and my Mediterranean Method in particular is gut-friendly.

When the Gut Barrier Is Injured

WHEN THE LINING of the intestinal tract is breached or injured—which happens when bad microbes overwhelm the gut—the gut lining becomes inflamed and permeable and starts to leak, allowing food, microbes, and waste (stool) from the gut into the bloodstream. This breakdown of the gut barrier is known as leaky gut syndrome, and it can trigger a cascade of health problems.

As foreign particles enter the bloodstream, the body responds with inflammatory compounds, and body-wide inflammation increases dramatically. The inflamed gut, with microbes passing across the gut lining, alerts the immune system to attack, causing

additional damage, and as systemic inflammation increases, this creates a vicious circle that is hard to stop.

In the short term, a leaky gut makes you achier, you might notice brain fog and decreased concentration, your energy drops, and you have increased bloating and other GI symptoms. If this is allowed to continue over the long term, it can trigger an autoimmune attack, with your immune system attacking your own tissues. Some autoimmune disorders resulting from leaky gut include inflammatory bowel disease, multiple sclerosis, thyroid disease, and psoriasis.

Over time, the harmful microbe

imbalance (known medically as dysbiosis) that results from leaky gut will lead to substantial weight gain, and the prolonged rise in inflammation increases your risk for heart disease and memory loss, as well.

Sadly, the leaky gut syndrome is common in people who follow the Standard American Diet with a lack of adequate fiber and an overload of sugar and refined carbs, all of which will cause inflammation and overgrowth of bad bacteria.

Some medications can also cause a leaky gut—in particular, antibiotics (discussed in detail shortly) and nonsteroidal anti-inflammatory drugs (NSAIDs). NSAIDs include over-the-counter medications, which may be sitting in your medicine cabinet now, such as ibuprofen, naproxen, and aspirin. There are prescription-strength NSAIDs, too, such as Celebrex, which is used to treat joint, tendon, and muscle aches. While NSAIDs do temporarily decrease joint pain and inflammation, they can also cause major gastrointestinal leaking and initiate leaky gut syndrome. My general rule with my patients is to avoid them and find alternative ways to address inflammation and relieve pain. (You'll find that eating an anti-inflammatory diet, such as the Mediterranean diet, goes a long way toward addressing the root cause!) If you must use NSAIDs, make it a rare occurrence—not more than five to ten days per year.

Avoid These Gut Microbiome Killers Now

THERE ARE TWO ways to support your gut health. The first step is to rid your system of compounds that deplete good bacteria. The next step is to restore and nourish friendly microbes, with help from the best diet on the planet. Before we move to gut-supporting nutrients that you can get from a Mediterranean diet, here are three common killers you should avoid.

1. ANTIBIOTICS

Just a single brief five-, seven-, or ten-day course of antibiotics can kill billions of gut microbes and disrupt the normal balance in your intestinal tract for months or even years. This is why I've been adamant with my clinic patients that they avoid taking antibiotics for colds, bronchitis, or intestinal symptoms that will likely resolve on their own.

Of course, antibiotics play a vital role when treating serious infections, such as pneumonia, cellulitis, or a kidney infection, but according to the Centers for Disease Control and Prevention (CDC), well over one-third of antibiotics prescribed in the United States are used inappropriately, including for minor illnesses that will resolve without any medical therapy. Always ask your physician if you can safely give an infection time to run its course before starting a round of antibiotics.

If you do need to start a course of antibiotic therapy, you should also start taking a probiotic supplement containing at least 25 to 50 billion bacteria, and continue taking it for several months (after your antibiotic prescription) to help restore normal gut microbes. And of course, following a Mediterranean diet is a great way to provide prebiotic fiber (from fibrous plant foods, which will be discussed later in this chapter), which encourages your gut bacteria to multiply and repopulate your intestinal tract.

2. WEED KILLERS

One of the most commonly used weed killers (herbicides) is the controversial product Roundup, a glyphosate compound used in agriculture throughout the United States and in other parts of the world. Not only does it exterminate weeds but also, when ingested by humans who eat foods sprayed with glyphosate (for instance, the grain fed to cattle, the wheat used in bread products, or conventionally grown produce), it also kills healthy gut bacteria. According to multiple studies, even trace quantities of glyphosate will deplete healthy gut microbes. There is also solid

evidence that consuming Roundup appears to increase cancer risk as well.

Because Roundup is so widely used, many agricultural products—from produce to meat and dairy—are potentially tainted by it. The only way to effectively avoid it is to buy certified organically grown foods which are raised without toxic chemical herbicides and pesticides. Disturbingly, in the United States, we use about 200 million pounds of this poison on our crops; while it is used in other parts of the world, some Mediterranean countries have taken legislative steps to reduce its use, and throughout the European Union there is an ongoing movement to ban it altogether, especially in France and Italy.

3. ARTIFICIAL SWEETENERS

The inventors of the chemical sweetener Splenda (sucralose) must have thought that they had struck gold—and given its popularity, they did. By attaching a chloride to a sugar molecule, they blocked the absorption of sugar across the intestinal tract. That's why when you consume this chlorinated sugar compound, you taste sweetness, but you don't absorb any calories.

In theory, it seems like the ideal way to allow people to consume sweet-tasting food products without the calories and impact on blood sugar levels. But in the same way that adding chlorine to water kills bacteria, combining chlorine with sugar kills some of the healthy bacteria in your gut. (What's great for a swimming pool is not great for your gut.)

It's not just chlorinated sugars that have a negative impact on the gut microbiome.

It turns out that other artificial sweeteners such as aspartame (NutraSweet and Equal) and saccharine (Sweet 'N Low) can work in a similar way, depleting good gut bacteria. One group of Israeli researchers have reported that artificial sweeteners enhance the populations of gut bacteria that are more efficient at pulling energy from our food and turning that energy into fat than in people who did not consume an artificial sweetener.

Interestingly, many European countries have called for artificial sweeteners to be banned, and their use has never reached the same widespread levels as in the United States. Mediterranean dwellers have an appetite for natural food sources (not substitutes conjured in a chemistry lab) and an abhorrence to the idea of artificial flavors. Their taste for great food has probably spared them from being harmed by excessive use of artificial sweeteners.

Use Diet to Prevent Disease

EAT A MEDITERRANEAN DIET TO SUPPORT YOUR GUT— AND PREVENT DISEASE

Supporting the gut and maintaining a strong gut barrier are essential to long-term good health, ensuring proper nutrient absorption, preventing leaky gut syndrome, and reducing inflammation. And, of course, the most important way to promote gut health is through diet.

When you support your gut through choosing the right foods, *you also protect your heart and brain*—but the reverse is true, as well. In a major 2017 meta-analysis published in the *Journal of the American Heart Association*, researchers concluded that a compound produced by gut bacteria seriously increased the risk of a major cardiovascular event, including heart attack and stroke. Individuals with high levels of TMAO (trimethylamine-N-oxide), a compound generated when gut bacteria metabolize an amino acid called carnitine (and to a lesser degree choline) were 62 percent more at risk for experiencing major adverse cardiovascular events and 63 percent more at risk for death of any cause.

A major source of carnitine is red meat—as some nutrition experts say, the redder the meat, the higher the carnitine. But individuals who follow a Mediterranean diet and eat lots of vegetables (whether they are omnivorous or vegetarian) have decreased production of TMAO. (Note: Carnitine, which is essential for building muscle mass, is also found in lower amounts in fish, poultry, and milk. Choline, found in eggs, liver, and peanuts, is important for brain health. But an excess of these two amino acids can lead to dangerously high levels of TMAO.)

It turns out that consuming more olive oil, red wine, and balsamic vinegar is one potential way to reduce TMAO production from gut bacteria. A true Mediterranean diet—a way of eating that I have been advocating for years—is rich with those gut-friendly foods and low in foods that not only hurt the microbiome (processed foods, sugars, bad fats) but also damage the heart.

To avoid a TMAO-related jump in cardiovascular disease risk, you have two options. Either you can go vegan and totally avoid carnitine and choline to prevent them from being converted to TMAO (though you'd eliminate two healthy nutrients), or much easier—and some would say healthier as you'll get some carnitine and choline—you can adopt a Mediterranean diet and eat more foods to support your gut. In particular, you'll be eating more prebiotic fiber and more probiotic foods with live microbes that will populate your gut.

PREBIOTICS AND PROBIOTICS

Prebiotics are sources of fiber that intestinal bacteria use as fuel. Prebiotics are all made of fiber, but not all types of fibers are prebiotics. Eating more prebiotic fiber will not only support your gut microbes but also improve cholesterol and blood sugar levels, and enhance blood pressure control as well.

One of the ways a traditional Mediterranean diet improves your gut microbiome is that it is an incredibly rich source of fiber that healthy gut microbes use as a food source. Without adequate fiber, your healthy gut bacteria die off. Some of the best sources of prebiotic fiber come from vegetables, fruits, beans, nuts, and whole grains—features of the Mediterranean diet.

There are a variety of technical terms that describe prebiotic fiber, including inulin, oligofructose, and glucomannan. Yet, far more practical is to identify foods that are loaded with prebiotic fiber so that you can eat and enjoy them more often. Some of the top sources of prebiotic fibers are:

- Artichokes (including Jerusalem artichokes), a great source of prebiotic fiber, especially inulin, which has been linked to better appetite control.

- Dandelion greens (native to the Mediterranean Sea), a bitter green that can be mixed and cooked with other greens, or added to mixed greens in a salad. It helps support healthy gut bacteria.

- Arugula, kale, radicchio, and mint. These are all classified as bitter greens as well, and eating a variety of them has a double benefit: They provide an excellent source of prebiotic fiber, but the bitterness also stimulates acid production in the stomach and improves digestion and nutrient absorption. Legumes, especially lentils and chickpeas, will also help with digestion.

- Garlic, onions, leeks, and shallots—also good for digestion.

- Asparagus—try eating spears raw or blanching them for maximum fiber.

- Apples, pears, oranges—my favorite fruits for prebiotic fiber.

- Jicama. Use it thinly sliced for dipping instead of chips or crackers.

- Oats and barley. If you eat whole grains, these have the highest inulin content and also happen to have the lowest glycemic load among whole grains (though barley contains gluten, so if you are gluten sensitive, avoid all products that contain barley).

- Konjac root (a thickener for sauces). This tuber is 40 percent glucomannan fiber, a highly viscous dietary fiber that promotes the growth of friendly bacteria in the colon.

- Nuts and seeds, especially almonds and pistachios.

- Cocoa powder, an often-overlooked source of fiber (and antioxidants). Try adding a tablespoon to your morning coffee—my version of a mocha—or in a smoothie.

Probiotics are live bacteria and microbes in a food source that help support a healthy gut. Though you won't see probiotic-rich fermented foods such as sauerkraut or miso on a list of traditional Mediterranean foods, you will find probiotic-rich dairy (detailed on pages 48–49), as well as olives and crunchy, savory pickled vegetables (known as *giardiniera* in Italy and served as antipasti; see my Marinated Mediterranean Olives and Vegetables, page 170). Some of the top sources of probiotics are:

- Yogurt

- Kefir

- Raw, unpasteurized cheese

- Olives (a fermented food)

- Pickled/marinated vegetables (fermented)

More Disease-Fighting Benefits

EVEN OLIVE OIL impacts the gut microbiota in a favorable way, according to several recent studies. In one, Italian researchers found evidence that olive oil consumption, which not only feeds healthy gut bacteria but also fights inflammation and oxidative stress, could reduce the risk of *colorectal cancer*.

The polyphenol content in olive oil, it appears, may disrupt interactions between gut microbiota that lay the groundwork for developing cancers. Though more research is needed, scientists are starting to explore the links between colorectal cancer—as well as other cancers—and the compounds in olive oil that may well have protective effects against this disease.

The Mediterranean diet also lowers your risk for *fatty liver*. Nearly 30 percent of the population has non-alcoholic fatty liver disease (NAFLD—also referred to as "fatty liver"), a result of poor blood sugar control, with excess sugars getting stored in the liver as fat. NAFLD increases the risk for serious liver damage, cirrhosis, Type 2 diabetes, and cardiovascular disease. Obesity and hepatic insulin resistance are the primary causes of fatty liver. Losing body fat clearly helps, and so does increasing insulin sensitivity. Researchers in Australia studied the impact of a Mediterranean diet and a low-fat diet on patients with fatty liver. Following a Mediterranean diet for just six weeks improved their insulin sensitivity and researchers also noted a significant reduction in fatty liver.

If You Have Gluten Sensitivity and Gut Inflammation

FOR PEOPLE WITH gluten sensitivity, eating gluten can cause major gut inflammation and leaky gut syndrome, along with a variety of non-GI symptoms. Since 20 percent of the United States population has been reported to have gluten sensitivity, an important question becomes: Who should go gluten-free?

Let's start by clarifying precisely what this substance is. Gluten is a protein found in all products made from wheat, rye, and barley. Wheat flour is by far the most prevalent source of gluten and is used throughout the food industry to manufacture thousands of processed foods. Gluten in flour provides texture, it helps dough rise during heating, and it creates a product that is fluffy and moist—all reasons that the food industry loves using it.

To our immune systems, gluten proteins look in some ways like human proteins—and for a significant number of people this molecular similarity can be disastrous. When a person has a reaction to gluten, his or her immune system will produce antibodies that attack gluten (which it considers a foreign invader), but unfortunately these same antibodies can also attack the person's gut lining, joints, sinuses, thyroid, skin, and brain.

This reaction is an example of autoimmunity, which is why gluten sensitivity is considered by many experts to be an autoimmune disease: If you're gluten sensitive and you consume gluten, then your body will make antibodies that attack and damage your own tissues. This is why autoimmune diseases can be both disabling and deadly, including multiple sclerosis and inflammatory bowel disease, which may be triggered by gluten.

Gluten sensitivity is vastly more serious than an ordinary food intolerance. Let's use lactose intolerance—one of the most common of the food intolerances—as a comparison. Lactase is the enzyme you need to digest milk sugar (lactose), and when you don't have lactase, consuming milk, ice cream, and other dairy products makes you gassy and bloated. For some people, it can also result in painful abdominal cramps. But other than some short-term annoying symptoms, eating dairy products with lactose doesn't kill you.

Gluten, however, is a different story. If you are gluten sensitive, every time you eat foods containing wheat, rye, or barley, your immune system "sees" the gluten protein and treats it like a foreign invader, making antibodies that go into attack mode as described here—except that your body is the very thing that's under attack. When you're gluten sensitive, even if you just eat it once every two weeks, you may have nonstop symptoms because the antibody attack is a relentless cycle. Eat it just once, and it has the potential to trigger your immune system into attacking your tissues for the next twenty to thirty days. The symptoms of gluten sensitivity include:

- Gastrointestinal issues: bloating, gassy, abdominal pain

- Brain fog, anxiety, or depression

- Achy joints

- Sinus congestion

- Fatigue

- Weight gain and resistant weight loss (i.e., you do everything right but still can't lose weight)

- Eczema and psoriasis rashes

If you're gluten sensitive, you can have all these symptoms or as few as one or two. At my clinic, I recommend either gluten laboratory testing or a gluten-free elimination diet trial for a minimum of three to four weeks for anyone with any of the chronic, unexplained symptoms as noted here.

Going gluten-free can be a challenge. Many people try to follow a gluten-free elimination diet and inadvertently eat foods with gluten, such as a condiment, a flavoring, or an ingredient in what otherwise seemed to be a gluten-free food (for example, a canned vegetable soup or broth, or any food item that doesn't list a gluten ingredient but somehow became contaminated with a gluten protein). In addition, according to some studies, so-labeled "gluten-free" crackers, breads, and snacks use flours that are, in fact, contaminated with gluten. Therefore they fail to go truly gluten-free.

At the urging of a patient, I tried going gluten-free myself—he wanted me to experience just how hard it really is—and I had to try three times before I made it totally gluten-free for at least one month. Of course, as a nutritionist and physician, I was able to avoid gluten entirely when I prepared my own food in my own kitchen. But when I have to eat out, like everyone else I'm at the mercy of the server who assures me the dish I'm ordering is "gluten-free." At a Japanese restaurant, for instance, the server swore the rice noodles were gluten-free. After I ate my meal, she returned to the table and apologized, having just learned the noodles I'd consumed contained wheat flour! At that point I'd gone twenty days gluten-free, but I had to start all over again the next day.

Clearly—and as my own experience shows—unless you are ultra-careful when you try a one-month gluten-free trial, testing is the way to go to confirm a diagnosis. But testing can also be a challenge because many doctors order an outdated blood test for gluten sensitivity. Known as tissue transglutaminase antibody, or tTG (also called TGG), this outdated test looks at antibodies against gluten protein, but often misses people with known gluten sensitivity. If the test is positive, you have confirmed gluten sensitivity; but the test can yield a false-negative result in people who have non-celiac gluten sensitivity. That's because your body breaks gluten down into many smaller allergenic protein particles, and more than 50 percent of the time you can react to these gluten metabolites (called gliadins), but not react to gluten protein itself. The standard test will then miss these smaller metabolite reactions in people with true gluten sensitivity.

In my clinic, we use a laboratory called Vibrant Wellness and a test called Wheat Zoomer, both of which test for both leaky gut syndrome and wheat antibodies. The problem is, of course, the expense, around $250 to $300 per test, and typically this isn't covered by medical insurance. Still, confirming that you are wheat sensitive means that you have a solution to potentially multiple chronic medical problems, so this testing can be well worth the expense.

In people with celiac disease, a gluten-triggered autoimmune disorder, the immune system attacks the gut and damages the small intestine. Many people in search of a reason for GI problems think that if they test negative for celiac disease they can eat gluten, but because of the possibility of false-negative results, and because it is possible to have gluten sensitivity without having celiac disease, that's not the case. In that instance, the antibodies may not destroy the gut lining, but they may attack and damage the brain and lead to neurodegenerative conditions such as multiple sclerosis. Gluten sensitivity, which brings about a constant state of body-wide inflammation, may also increase the risk for lymphoma and lead to thyroid problems, and at minimum it can cause GI issues, weight gain, skin rashes (such as eczema), body aches and pains, and chronic fatigue.

If you or a loved one suffers from any of the symptoms related to gluten sensitivity listed here, I strongly encourage you to either follow a totally gluten-free trial for at least thirty days or have definitive testing for gluten sensitivity.

Gluten and the Mediterranean Diet

IF YOU TEST positive for gluten, then give it up completely. Don't limit your intake—avoid it 100 percent, as your long-term health depends on it. Do a careful search for gluten-containing foods and products; it is hiding in many places you may not suspect. Fortunately, because so many people are demanding gluten-free options, you'll find more and more options, not only in your supermarket but also when you go out for a meal. Just be vigilant, ask lots of questions, and read labels very carefully; gluten sensitivity means that even trace amounts of contamination may set off inflammation. You might consider taking gluten digestive enzymes (a supplement), which can help you digest small, occasional amounts of gluten contamination. (For more information on gluten digestive enzymes, visit www.drmasley.com/resources.)

You can follow my Mediterranean Method and stay completely gluten-free. The majority of the 50-plus recipes are all gluten-free, and the couple of recipes that do include a gluten option (such as pasta) provide a gluten-free alternative. Here are a few steps that are important to succeed.

- Give up wheat, barley, and rye. That includes bread and pasta made with wheat flour (which have a fairly high glycemic load and should be limited by anyone following the Mediterranean Method).

- Instead of seeking out commercially available gluten-free flour products (many of which are processed foods), avoid the majority of flour—after all, it is mostly a refined carb similar to sugar and you don't need it. If you want a gluten-free chip, bread, or pasta, it is available, likely using a combination of chickpea, potato, quinoa, or rice flour, but there are so many other great foods you can eat that you will find you don't miss them. If you do eat gluten-free products, take a gluten digestive enzyme to help cover you for any trace contamination.

- Purchase an inexpensive spiralizer and enjoy fresh "spaghetti" made from zucchini and other gut-friendly fibrous vegetables.

- Make sure to use gluten-free condiments and dressings. Soy sauce is not a part of the traditional Mediterranean diet, but in any event avoid this gluten-contaminated food—use tamari instead.

- Instead of store-bought dressing, make your own flavor-packed dressings. Why not simply go for a dressing or vinaigrette like the one on page 185, or just try a squirt of lemon juice or balsamic vinegar, a drizzle of olive oil, and some herbs?

When Dairy Causes Gut Issues

Lactose intolerance is likely the world's #1 food intolerance, impacting more than two-thirds of people on the planet and causing a variety of GI symptoms, including abnormal flatulence, cramping, and abdominal pain. The major source for lactose (milk sugar) is milk, ice cream, cream, and soft cheeses—which by tradition are not part of a Mediterranean diet. Historically there was no refrigeration to preserve these perishables; instead, there was (and still is) yogurt, kefir, and hard cheeses that didn't require cold storage, and these dairy foods have very little lactose. In fact, you can easily avoid most lactose and follow a Mediterranean eating plan.

Milk protein allergy, much more serious than lactose intolerance, is far less common but still impacts millions of people. If you are sensitive to dairy protein, then consuming it will cause GI inflammation and can lead to leaky gut, just as gluten impacts those with gluten sensitivity.

The only real solution for dairy protein sensitivity is to avoid all dairy products. As an alternative to yogurt and kefir, you can buy fermented coconut milk, almond milk yogurt, and cashew nut milk, and substitute any of these as a yogurt alternative. Finding a substitute for grated hard cheese, such as Parmigiano Reggiano, is more challenging. Soy cheese doesn't melt the way hard cheese does nor does it provide the same flavor.

If dairy doesn't agree with you, the best, gut-friendliest option is to skip the grated cheese. It's not worth it, nor is it essential, as we're just talking about a small quantity. Try chopped or slivered nuts as a garnish instead.

You Can Heal Your Gut

IF YOU HAVE symptoms suggesting dysbiosis and/or leaky gut syndrome, you can heal your intestinal tract to stop the leaking and repopulate your gut with gut-healthy microbes. Focus on these five key goals that I share with my patients:

1. Eat at least 10 servings (more than 30 grams) of fiber per day, preferably from vegetables, fruits, beans, and nuts.

2. Eat 1–2 servings of probiotic-rich foods daily.

3. Take a probiotic supplement with at least 25–50 billion live microbes per day. Ideally this will have a balance of healthy bacteria and fungi to restore a healthy gut microbiome.

4. Take a glutamine supplement, 2,000 to 3,000 mg per day.

5. Follow an elimination diet and avoid all gluten and dairy for at least 30 days.

Now you know how my Mediterranean Method can help you lose weight, prevent heart disease, protect your brain health, and heal your gut. It can also help you add years to your life and turn back the clock on aging, as you'll see in the next chapter.

Mediterranean Your Way: For Gut Health

- A Mediterranean diet is an effective way to help you maintain or regain good gut health—and, of course, overall health.

- When you follow the Mediterranean Method, you'll naturally get plenty of prebiotic fiber as well as probiotic-rich foods, and you'll avoid foods that can weaken your gut barrier and cause inflammation.

- Address any issues you may have with gut-damaging gluten—if you suspect you have sensitivity, work with your doctor to get accurate testing and help following a carefully monitored elimination diet.

- Beyond food, supplement as needed to heal and support good gut health.

7

THE MEDITERRANEAN METHOD FOR LONGEVITY

Americans have an average life span of 78.7 years, according to recent statistics from the CDC and data from the National Vital Statistics System. By 2030, it is expected to rise—but only by about one year, to 79.8 years. Of course, it's impossible to predict how long any one of us will live. But consider this: Rather than aim for a big number, why not aim for a big number of healthy, disease-free years? It's one thing to live into your 80s and 90s, but if you are frail, sick, and depressed about the state of your declining health—not for years but for decades—then living to a "ripe old age" doesn't seem very appealing.

Considering all you've learned about the benefits of a Mediterranean diet and the Mediterranean Method, it won't come as a surprise that people in Italy, France, and especially Spain live on average an additional two to four years more than Americans. And they enjoy these additional years living *well*—that is, without our epidemic levels of illness, disability, and obesity.

A wealth of research points to this fact: People who follow a Mediterranean diet have the longest life span and best health on the planet—so much so that the World Health Organization has created guidelines for *everyone* on the planet to follow a Mediterranean-style eating plan; whether you live in Europe, the United States, or elsewhere, the closer you adhere to these dietary recommendations, the longer you live and the less disease you have.

The Longevity Lifestyle

The United States has been considered the land of plenty for generations. But it's not necessarily the land of long-lived, healthy people. When a government agency recently released its annual ranking of countries with the longest life expectancies, the United States wasn't even in the top 30. The United States came in at 43—well behind dozens of countries that don't approach our per capita income, but that leave us behind when it comes to long lives, free of chronic disease.

One of those countries is Spain, where the people enjoy one of the longest life expectancies among all of the Mediterranean countries, living to an average age of 82—about four years longer than the average American. (The world-famous PREDIMED study on the benefits of a traditional Mediterranean diet, cited earlier, was based in Spain.) Besides traveling through inland Spain, more recently for this book I have sailed along the entire Spanish coastline, visiting ports and villages along the way, sampling local foods, shopping in markets, sampling regional foods, and cooking with local ingredients (and developing recipes to share with you).

In these ancient Spanish coastal communities, even as modern life has taken hold, they still follow many aspects of a Mediterranean lifestyle, something that most certainly accounts for their longevity. Here are seven reasons why people live longer in Spain than they do in the United States, and why that trend will continue. In fact, by the year 2030, the people of Spain are projected to have the longest life span of any country in the world!

1. *They follow a Mediterranean diet closely*, with more vegetables, fruits, beans, and seafood, with lots of spices and herbs, and of course, plenty of olive oil. They enjoy fresh fruit daily, although one area even the Spanish need to improve upon is to eat more green leafy vegetables daily. Only half the population reportedly eats a green leafy vegetable every day, but that is double what we consume in the United States. As I tell my patients, eating just one serving of green leafy vegetables daily makes your brain eleven years younger than that of someone who doesn't eat them.

2. *They prepare their own food and avoid processed items.* Most Spanish people tend to purchase real food made with pure, basic ingredients, which makes their food taste better and exposes them to fewer toxins and hormones in their food than we are. They also cook their meals, instead of buying prepared meals, and as most people eat this way, the cost for vegetables, fruits, beans, nuts, olive oil, and even poultry and seafood is far less expensive than what we pay for the same types of food in

the United States. They do have prepared food in grocery stores, but it is relatively more expensive than in the United States, making it far less appealing.

3. *They are active.* They walk to work, to shop for groceries, and to get around the neighborhood. They are far less dependent on their cars. In addition to just

---

Living Long, Staying Strong: Lessons from Japan

The aim should be not just to live long but also to remain healthy. In Japan, home to the Blue Zone dwellers of Okinawa, the average life expectancy is over 85 years. In addition, the Japanese have much lower levels of obesity, heart disease, and other ailments compared to Westerners, especially Americans. They don't just live longer than most people on the planet; they also have more years of good health.

Early on, I touched on a few commonalities between the Okinawan diet and that of Mediterranean dwellers (see page 20). More specifically:

- *The traditional diet in Okinawa (and elsewhere in Japan) relies heavily on vegetables.*

- *They also eat an abundance of fruits, beans, and unprocessed carbohydrates.*

- *They consume seafood often.*

- *Traditionally they don't use olive oil, yet they use oils with a similar high ratio of mono/polyunsaturated fats, plus a diet rich in long-chain omega-3 fats and less saturated fats.*

- *They drink lots of tea, and their alcohol intake overall is fairly moderate.*

- *They eat very little red meat.*

Like the Mediterranean Method, the Japanese way of eating features a low glycemic load, with foods rich in phytonutrients and antioxidants that decrease levels of inflammation. If you don't live in Japan, however, eating an Okinawan-style diet is not easy to do. Consuming traditional Japanese fish dishes, pickled vegetables, and natto on a regular basis would be a challenge—not just because of sourcing and preparing these staples but also because their tastes and flavors don't appeal to everyone. Following a Mediterranean diet, however, is quite doable.

Here's an interesting side note on Japan's high life-expectancy ranking. No doubt their longevity statistics are bolstered by much lower levels of chronic disease. The country has dominated the top spots for life expectancy, but in recent years their longevity has decreased a bit. Some researchers suggest this slip is because more Japanese are eating like Westerners—that is, like Americans, with a taste for processed food and fast food. It could be that following a traditional diet is becoming harder in modern Japan, especially in its fast-paced cities.

walking as a mode of transportation, more than 60 percent of Spaniards report exercise beyond walking. Everywhere I have traveled in Spain, I see people jogging, bicycling, boating, swimming, and scuba diving. The Spanish spend more time outdoors, and they even eat their meals outside, soaking up some sunshine and making more vitamin D.

4. *They have one-third less obesity than we have.* Only 23.8 percent of the population was listed as obese in 2016 statistics, compared to 36.2 percent of Americans (a number that continues to inch upward). Of course, this is largely due to their food choices and activity levels.

5. *Far more people in Spain have access to good-quality health care.* Only 1 percent of the Spanish people report that their medical needs were not met, compared

to the United States, where, according to the Congressional Budget Office in 2019, 29 million Americans do not have health insurance. Spaniards are likely not as sick as Americans in part because their lifestyle offers built-in preventive health care!

6. *In Spain, eating is a pleasure.* Unlike far too many Americans, people don't eat as often alone in front of a TV or at their desk. They socialize over meals, and enjoy food with family and friends.

7. *Overall, Spaniards generally seem happy.* In fact, they have one of the lowest depression and suicide rates in the world.

You could consider this list a prescription for a good life—it's no wonder the Spaniards live such long, healthy lives. Wherever you live, the Mediterranean Method can offer a pathway for you to do so, as well.

How a Mediterranean Diet Can Add Healthy Years to Your Life

ONE OF THE best measures of aging itself might be telomere length. Telomeres are the tips at the end of our cellular DNA strands, and they are essential for normal cell division and replication. Think of telomeres as having a function similar to those plastic tips at the

end of your shoelaces that protect the string from unraveling and breaking down.

As we age, our telomere length naturally shortens. But shortening of telomeres is also associated with injury, as well as life-ending disease, including cancer and heart disease. Once the protective telomeres wear away, cells essentially die off; some cell death is inevitable with normal aging, but the cells die before their time if disease sets in. In genetic studies that have compared how closely people follow a Mediterranean diet, researchers have found that the greater the adherence to the diet, the less telomere shortening that occurs. Essentially, this means that a Mediterranean diet can stop what amounts to accelerated aging triggered by disease.

You've already learned how the Mediterranean Method can work for weight loss, and how it can help to guard against heart disease and memory loss, the two most prevalent, life-threatening diseases facing the Western world today. But those aren't the only conditions it can address. The Mediterranean Method also helps prevent metabolic syndrome (including high blood sugar levels/insulin resistance, with or without progression to Type 2 diabetes), high levels of inflammation, and cancer. Let's look at how.

The Mediterranean Method and Reversing Metabolic Syndrome

YOUR METABOLISM REFERS to how efficiently you process energy at the cellular level, or to put it another way, what your body does with the food you eat. Ideally, and with the help of insulin, if you consume and absorb the nutrients your body requires and you're physically active, your cells will burn some of the energy you get from food when your body exerts itself, and store some energy for later use. But, when this metabolic process goes awry—usually because of eating excessive refined carbohydrates that send blood sugar levels on a roller-coaster ride and confuse the insulin response—this energy equilibrium is destroyed.

You can develop a serious condition known as metabolic syndrome (also referred to as syndrome X or pre-diabetes), a constellation of risk factors for heart disease and diabetes including:

1. An expanding waistline (more than a 40-inch waist circumference in men and more than 35 inches in women)

2. Elevated blood pressure (higher than 130/85)

3. Low levels of "good" HDL cholesterol (lower than 40 mg/dL for men, and lower than 50 mg/dL for women)

4. Elevated triglyceride levels (equal to or higher than 150 mg/dL)

5. High fasting blood sugar levels (equal to or higher than 100 mg/dL—note that this is often the last sign to occur and you may have pre-diabetes for years before this number is elevated)

6. Elevated inflammation levels (hs-CRP level greater than 1.0)—as measured by a high-sensitivity C-reactive protein blood test.

If you have any three of these criteria, then you qualify for a medical diagnosis of metabolic syndrome and pre-diabetes. If you have only one or two of these signs, you should still be alarmed: If you continue on the same path, you will likely progress and soon you will have more signs of this disorder. (Note: Some medical resources only list the first five risk factors; inflammation, the sixth sign, is extremely significant and it's a risk factor that I and many other experts now include.)

Elevated blood sugar levels on their own accelerate all aspects of aging. Sugar in your bloodstream will sugarcoat your proteins and make them more susceptible to damage. High sugar levels raise inflammation, causing irritation to your joints, arteries, brain, and many other organs.

Even mildly elevated blood sugar levels and levels in the top range of normal (a normal fasting blood sugar level is less than 100 mg/dL) increase your risk for arterial plaque growth and heart disease, dementia, obesity, kidney disease, future diabetes, and cancer. High blood sugar levels lead to insulin resistance, which promotes weight gain,

death of brain cells and brain shrinkage, and growth of arterial plaque. Besides being triggered by eating too much sugar and foods with a high glycemic load, high blood sugar worsens when a person doesn't get enough physical activity, drinks too much alcohol, and fails to get adequate dietary fiber (typically it is from a combination of several of these issues).

The low-glycemic Mediterranean Method, however, may help to reverse metabolic syndrome. In the PREDIMED study, nearly 7,000 subjects with either multiple risk factors for heart disease or metabolic syndrome were randomized to either a Mediterranean diet with extra olive oil intake, or a Mediterranean diet with extra nut intake, or a control group following a standard low-fat diet, and were followed an average of 4.8 years.

At entry, 3,392 participants already had metabolic syndrome and, during the study, 958 (28.2 percent) were able to reverse this condition. Those following the two arms of the Mediterranean diet were 28 to 35 percent more likely to have reversed this problem than those following the low-fat diet. However, of the 960 subjects who developed metabolic syndrome during the study, the risk of developing this disorder was the same whether they followed one of the Mediterranean diet interventions or not.

For me, this last result is a clear sign that we can *improve* on the standard Mediterranean diet by using the low-glycemic twist offered by the Mediterranean Method. It's true that the traditional Mediterranean diet has been followed by farmers and fishermen for centuries, but we live in a modern world with less activity and more chemical exposure, where servings of bread, pasta, rice, and too many carbs (including too many "healthy" whole grains) provide an excessive glycemic load that sets people up for metabolic syndrome.

Over the last 25 years, most of my patients with metabolic syndrome have been able to reverse it, largely through following an early version of the Mediterranean Method.

I also worked with a group of my patients who had uncontrolled diabetes, most of whom were on medications, some receiving daily insulin shots. I believed then (and now) that the standard American diet and their inactive lifestyle was what was killing them. We focused on the right foods to add, the right activity, and how to meet their nutrient needs. I even did cooking demos for the group and gave them recipes. (I can't emphasize enough what a difference it makes when you take charge of your meals and snacks!)

Within six months, more than half the group (those who followed my program the closest) were off all their diabetic medications and had normal blood sugar levels—they no longer had Type 2 diabetes. The rest of the group improved their blood sugar control—the closer they followed my plan, the more they improved. I did caution my patients that if they reverted to their old ways, they would backslide toward dangerous blood sugar levels and all the problems that come with it.

But here's the take-away: I've helped thousands of patients totally reverse metabolic syndrome and Type 2 diabetes, and bring blood sugar back under control through lifestyle changes—including the right food. And the theme I've used from the very beginning has been a low-glycemic-load version of the traditional Mediterranean diet—food that is a pleasure to make and eat—with extra activity and some form of proactive stress management.

It's the Mediterranean Method.

The Mediterranean Method and Reducing Inflammation

INFLAMMATION IS ANOTHER cause of accelerated aging and a decrease in life span. The word "inflammation" is rooted in the Latin word for "ignite"—and it's true that when your tissues are inflamed, they do feel hot (on fire) and sore. Pain, heat, redness, swelling, and loss of function are signs of inflammation, the body's biological response to an assault from an infection or injury.

In the short term, inflammation is the body's way of protecting itself. Yet the longer inflammation lasts, the more potential harm it can cause. If your joints are chronically inflamed, you get arthritis. If your lungs are inflamed, you develop asthma. If your brain is constantly inflamed, it will—ironically—slowly shrink over time. If your arteries are inflamed, you'll grow arterial plaque at an accelerated rate. If your gut—the #1 source of body-wide inflammation—is inflamed, your whole body can be at risk.

In my clinic, we measure systemic inflammation with a blood test called high-sensitivity C-reaction protein (hs-CRP). This is a test of a compound produced by the liver and a general barometer reading for how much systemic inflammation you have. An hs-CRP level less than 1.0 is normal, less than 0.5 is excellent, and more than 3.0 puts you at high risk for a cardiovascular event. Keep in mind that if you have an acute illness (even a cold) or a recent injury, inflammation is often

Sara Gottfried, MD, on the Mediterranean Diet

Brain Body Diet *author Sara Gottfried, MD, tells me that she especially appreciates the connection between a Mediterranean diet and a reduced risk of depression. Depression can take a toll at any age, even as you enter your "golden years." Combined with a lack of physical activity and a nutrient-poor diet, depression impacts your quality of life and your overall health—and it may even shorten your life span. But when you follow the Mediterranean Method you are taking steps to protect against that risk. "Consuming olive oil, fish, fruits, vegetables, nuts, legumes, poultry, and unprocessed, pastured meat—they are all associated with reduced depression risk and improved depression scores," she reminds us.*

To boost longevity, Sara suggests an intermittent fast: eating all food within an eight-hour window and abstaining for the other 16 at least one to two days per week, or for some people every day. Like me, she thinks it's best to go easy on whole grains, and suggests your brain and your body will benefit if you replace them with more vegetables.

part of the healing process, which is why I recommend that you don't measure your inflammation levels if you have had a cold, injury, or surgery in the last 30-plus days.

Fortunately, the Mediterranean diet is loaded with *high-potency, anti-inflammatory foods—in particular, extra-virgin olive oil and many Mediterranean herbs.* All the colorful plant pigments in vegetables and fruits also block inflammation. Nourish your gut—and your entire body—with the low-glycemic-load Mediterranean Method and you'll head off inflammation at the source, and the accelerated aging that comes with it.

Studies have shown that in people prone to inflammation (such as those with an underlying autoimmune disorder like rheumatoid arthritis), consuming extra-virgin olive oil will turn off inflammatory genes, lower hs-CRP levels, and reduce joint pain. But eating more refined carbs and sugar, especially if consumed with saturated fat sources from animal protein (for example, a bacon-cheeseburger), will increase the inflammatory pathways and cause more joint pain and other symptoms of inflammation. The combination of eating fatty animal protein and refined carbs causes far more inflammation than does eating either one by itself.

When you zero in on the dietary components that trigger inflammation—bad fats and sugar—it makes sense that the low-glycemic-load Mediterranean Method is the most effective way to put out these flames.

The Mediterranean Method and Decreasing Your Risk for Cancer

THE EVIDENCE IS overwhelming that if you follow a Mediterranean eating plan, you can lower your risk for cancer:

- Multiple scientific studies have shown that the closer you follow a Mediterranean diet, the lower your risk for many cancers, including breast, colon, prostate, uterus, throat, liver, and bladder cancers.

- Perhaps the largest of these recent, scientific meta-analyses included eighty-three separate publications and over 2 million combined subjects. Researchers were able to show that if you developed cancer and you followed a Mediterranean diet, you would be less likely to die from cancer and less likely to have a breast or colon cancer recurrence.

- For those who've survived cancer, similar studies have shown that following a Mediterranean diet can help them live longer (as compared to survivors who don't).

- Other recent publications showed that in northern Italy, women who followed a Mediterranean diet closely had 51 percent less chance of developing endometrial (uterine) cancer. In Switzerland, adhering to a Mediterranean diet decreased the risk for breast cancer. And researchers in Italy showed a 34 percent reduction in bladder cancer in those who came closest to following the diet.

- Olive-oil consumption has been shown by itself to reduce your risk for several cancers, including the colon, breast, and prostate, and to diminish the growth of colon polyps. Not only is olive oil rich in healthy fats but it also has a variety of phenolic compounds that lower inflammation, decrease oxidation, and have direct anti-cancer effects.

- Eating more vegetables and fruits consistently has been shown to lower the risk for many cancers (especially epithelial and GI tract cancers). Part of the benefit comes from eating fiber, and fruits and vegetables provide many antioxidant and anti-inflammatory compounds that reduce cancer risk.

Here's another cancer-reducing feature: The Mediterranean diet limits the use of red meat, and avoids processed deli meats. Multiple studies have shown that decreasing red meat intake will reduce cancer rates, especially from consuming deli meats and nitrosamine-laced products, like commercially produced bacon.

Conversely, eating refined grains will *increase* the risk of several cancers. A jump in fasting blood sugar levels increases insulin growth factor, a hormone related to insulin that has the potential to act as a fertilizer to promote the growth of many types of cancer. This makes my low-glycemic-load Mediterranean Method especially effective at lowering cancer risk.

It's Time to Quit Tobacco

Since we're discussing cancer, I must call out a non-dietary risk factor that accounts for 40 percent of all cancers in the United States: tobacco use. If you want to avoid cancer, avoid tobacco products. If you smoke or otherwise use tobacco, you'll undo all the benefits of even the healthiest diet on earth. If you need help quitting, please work with your healthcare provider to get help. There are many new behavioral modification programs and twenty-first-century treatments and medications that make it easier than before to walk away from this life-shortening habit.

Alcohol and Longevity

DOES ALCOHOL HELP you live longer, or does it shorten your life?

Moderate consumption of red wine in a Mediterranean diet is associated with good health, including protective benefits that lower the risk of cardiovascular disease, and multiple studies have shown that drinking modest amounts of alcohol can extend the life span, while consuming excess alcohol will shorten it.

But the relationship between alcohol and disease, especially cancer, is more complicated. First, some cancers are impacted by alcohol consumption and some are not. And second, we have to distinguish between total alcohol intake and type of alcohol.

If we include studies that look at total alcohol intake (hard liquor, beer, and wine combined), the conclusion seems to be this: The more alcohol you drink, the greater your risk for cancer, especially with excessive alcohol consumption (more than 4 servings per day). But keep in mind, modest intake (1–2 servings per day for women and 2–3 servings per day for men) lowers your risk for heart disease and diabetes, and this modest consumption also increases your life span.

When we separate types of alcohol and risk for cancer, we see a different story, as hard liquor, beer, and wine have different effects on different forms of cancer.

The higher your intake of hard liquor, the higher your risk for most types of cancer. Beer has a similar linear relationship with cancer, although a few types of cancers, such as kidney cancer, are reduced with moderate beer consumption but not with hard liquor. For kidney cancer, especially for women, modest wine consumption is associated with a lower risk for cancer.

In particular aggressive advanced forms of prostate cancer, after analyzing data on more than 2,000 patients, researchers have shown that higher beer intake, and very likely greater hard liquor intake, increases the risk for advanced or aggressive prostate cancer. In contrast, moderate wine consumption decreases the risk for prostate cancer.

Similarly, for gastrointestinal cancers, moderate wine consumption (defined as 1–3 servings per day) decreases the risk for these types of cancer. Both beer and liquor show a linear increasing risk the more alcohol that is consumed, starting at even one serving per day.

Overall, modest wine intake (1–2 servings per day for women and 2–3 servings per day for men), especially red wine, is associated with a slightly reduced risk for several forms of cancer. However, if you consume more than 3 servings per day, drinking any type of alcohol, including wine, is associated with an increased risk for cancer.

RED OR WHITE?

You'll find both red and white wines along the Mediterranean, although red wine is associated with more health benefits than white, probably because of the stronger concentrations of polyphenols (antioxidant compounds) found in the dark reds and purples of the grape skins.

Red wine polyphenols are a complex mixture of flavonoids (such as anthocyanins and flavan-3-ols) and nonflavonoids (such as resveratrol, cinnamates, and gallic acid). It's the biochemical behavior of these red wine compounds that makes a difference. They act as potent antioxidants as they reduce LDL "bad" cholesterol oxidation, modulate cell signaling pathways (allowing our cells to "talk" to each other clearly and perform their specialized functions), and reduce the clumping of blood platelets, lowering the chances of an arterial blockage.

Red wine contains about ten times more of these valuable polyphenols than white wine. During the making of red wine, in a process called maceration, the polyphenol-packed red–purple grape skins (as well as the seeds and stems) soak with the juice of the grape for varying periods of time (depending on the wine being produced) before they are removed prior to bottling.

BEFORE YOU POUR

It can be a challenge to untangle all the latest data, but if you drink alcohol and you're wondering how it impacts your longevity, here are the key points to keep in mind:

- Moderate wine consumption lowers your risk for cancer and is associated with many health benefits, including a longer life span and more healthy years.

- In moderation, red wine (which has a low glycemic load and works well with the Mediterranean Method) is the healthiest form of alcohol to consume, although having more than 3 servings per day is more harmful than beneficial.

- White wine has less benefit than red wine, but clearly more than other forms of alcohol. Beer and hard liquor have far less overall benefits than wine, and consuming them generally increases your risk for cancer.

The Mediterranean Method can help you prevent—and even reverse—life-shortening risk factors. But there's more to it than food, as I've been suggesting all along. It's a whole lifestyle.

I opened this chapter with a discussion on life expectancy rates and how the United States doesn't top any lists for longevity. But here's an interesting new finding. It seems that living to be 100 is on the rise among Americans (though minuscule compared to Blue Zones like Sardinia and Japan). In 1995, when the Boston University School of Medicine started the New England Centenarian Study (NECS), there was one centenarian for every 10,000 people; now it's one in 5,000. No doubt some of this is due to advances in medicine, biotechnology, and health care.

But again, the objective of the game of life isn't simply to live longer than everyone else.

It should be to live longer with more happy, healthy years at the end. And that's where overall lifestyle comes in. As the New England Centenarian Study reports, those Americans who live—in relative good health—to 100-plus years of age have found ways to handle stress well, are optimistic and outgoing, and have strong social connections. That sounds a lot like the Mediterranean attitude.

"I feel younger!"—Dave's Mediterranean Method Story

WHEN DAVE FIRST CAME TO SEE ME AT 60, he felt old before his time and tired, prepared to retire early—and quite depressed at the prospect of doing so. But Dave agreed to give my method a try and switch out the processed foods that had been a part of his diet for too long, choosing instead real, whole foods—Mediterranean-inspired fresh foods that he enjoyed much more than what he'd been eating before. Dave also incorporated plenty of daily activity into his life, which gave him much more energy and improved his state of mind. Eventually, he lost 25 pounds, his fitness level improved dramatically, and his brain processing speed improved by 50 percent. Now, at age 71, Dave is still working and traveling internationally. "I don't feel old!" Dave told me. "I feel younger, and I'm fitter, trimmer, sharper and have more energy than when I was 60!" The Mediterranean Method transformed him—and *added healthy years to his life.*

The Mediterranean Diet: Make It Yours

- Enjoy foods on the Mediterranean diet that have been proven to help to extend a healthy life span—especially olive oil, plant foods, and moderate red wine consumption.

- Follow the Mediterranean Method to blunt three of the biggest risk factors that cause accelerated aging and can cut your life short: metabolic syndrome, inflammation, and cancer.

- Live well, live longer: If you smoke (use tobacco products) and drink too much, chances are you're taking years off your life. Please get help if you need to quit tobacco or moderate your alcohol intake.

8

BRINGING THE MEDITERRANEAN DIET HOME

It's not just the wonderful food that makes the Mediterranean diet so appealing—and makes you younger, trimmer, fitter, mentally sharper, and prevents heart disease. As I've explained throughout this book, it's the entire lifestyle: how Mediterranean dwellers move through their day (and move, they do); how they cherish family, socialize with friends, and connect with the greater community; how they shop, prepare and share their meals; how they manage everyday stress, yet still manage to have fun every day.

One advantage to our fast-paced, hyper-connected, high-tech existence is this: In today's world, it is possible to bring the best of the Mediterranean diet and lifestyle right into your own home—and your kitchen—no matter where you live, even as you put your own stamp on it. You can sit down at your computer and order ingredients, watch a cooking demonstration, and learn how to finally flip an omelet or grow your own herbs, or walk into a suburban grocery store and find the makings of a Mediterranean meal, including foods, herbs, and spices imported from half a world away.

My Mediterranean Method was developed with *you* in mind, and *your* reality—not someone who lives in a French fishing village and can stroll down to the local market and buy today's catch for tonight's dinner. I know from decades of treating my patients and meeting people with health issues all across the country that everyone faces personal hurdles that can get in the way of making a change for the better.

Maybe you work long hours or have lots of free time; . . . care for a small child (or an elderly parent); . . . live in an apartment building with little outdoor space, . . . or in a suburb with no sidewalks and lots of cars. It doesn't matter what you do or where you are. If you are ready to let the Mediterranean Method change your life, all you need is one desire: to feel good inside and out, to be happier, and to add more healthy years to your life. That—and one more thing: . . . some practical know-how to get you started.

Here are my tips on how you can optimize your health as you bring the Mediterranean home—wherever home may be.

CUISINE, COCINA, CUCINA, KOUZÍNA: THE MOST IMPORTANT WORD IS "KITCHEN"

If you're looking for a small way to make a big change in your health—and to do something very Mediterranean—prepare your own food at home. As many times a week as you can manage. Fix breakfast. Make lunch. Pull together a nice dinner and make it from unprocessed food. Starting on page 164, you'll find more than 50 recipes that I developed to help you get started. The recipes are designed to be easy to make, with ingredients that you can find at your local store, and that your friends and family will love. Please don't tell me your kitchen is too cramped or your stove is too unreliable—because I created and tested almost all these recipes in the compact galley kitchen aboard a sailboat! You can do this—and when you can't, plan ahead. Get good at cooking things in batches, freezing extras, and having some essential fresh items as well as pantry staples on hand. (You'll also find a list of kitchen tips, pantry essentials, and shopping suggestions later in this chapter.)

EAT MINDFULLY

Mindless eating—it's almost a national pastime in the United States. Eating fast. Eating on the run. Eating in front of the TV or at your desk. Eating alone. As far as I know, the American expression "grab-and-go" does not translate into any other language! It's time to slow down and eat the Mediterranean way: mindfully, with care, and with joy.

Try these tips:

- *Declare your space for eating.* Put your food on a plate and dedicate a place to sit and eat it (not in front of the television, not in the car, not in front of the computer, and not at your desk). Better yet, as often as you can, sit with a loved one you want to spend time with or with a wider circle of friends and family. Look at your food and your surroundings before you start your meal, and allow yourself to get ready to enjoy your food.

- *Before you take your first bite, stop and ask yourself this question: "Are you hungry?"* Are you about to eat because you need fuel, or because you are upset, bored, or stressed out? Those reasons don't mean you shouldn't eat, but be very clear "why" you are eating, or you risk uncontrolled eating (especially if you're stressed), and subsequently, regret.

- *Visualize, smell, taste, and feel the food in your mouth, including each and every bite.* Before your first bite, look at the presentation of your food. Is your plate colorful, and do the portions match your appetite? As you slip your first bite across your lips, how does the food taste? Can you smell the food as you eat it? What is the texture like in your mouth? Switch from one item on your plate to another, and appreciate the difference between each bite. It is hoped that first bite tastes

Picking a Multivitamin

You should be able to meet most of your needs for heart-boosting magnesium, vitamin K, and potassium with food alone if you follow a Mediterranean eating plan (see Chapter 4 for detailed information), but I generally recommend you add a quality multivitamin for other nutrients such as mixed folates and chromium, sufficient amounts of which are more difficult to get through your food. Also, depending upon the amount of vitamin D in your multivitamin, you may need an additional source.

Be aware that you get what you pay for—cheap supplements from chain drugstores generally contain inferior forms of vitamins and minerals that your body can't absorb and use properly. Beyond price, here's another clue about quality: Acceptable multivitamins are usually at least two pills. The reason? It's impossible to compress adequate amounts of certain nutrients into a single small pill. The four brands I trust most are Designs for Health, Thorne Research, Metagenics, and ProThera (available online or through your health-care provider). Here is the information I share with patients who want to know what to look for—and what to avoid—when purchasing a multivitamin. (For more detailed information on multi-vitamin ingredients as well as sources that meet these criteria, visit www.drmasley.com /resources.) Be sure to look for these key ingredients when choosing a multivitamin:

- **Folacin or 5-MTHF (mixed folates)**—*not only folic acid*

- **Mixed carotenoids**—*not solely beta-carotene*

- **Mixed tocopherols/tocotrienols**—*not just alpha tocopherol, and most important are delta and gamma tocotrienols*

- **Protein-bound minerals (malates, glycinates)**—*not oxides (like magnesium oxide)*

- **Zinc-to-copper ratio of 20 or more**

- **Organic copper (copper glycinate)**—*not inorganic copper*

- **Chromium**—*at least 400 mcg*

- **Vitamin B$_{12}$ (cobalamin)**—*at least 100 mcg*

- **Vitamin D**—*at least 1,000 IUs and preferably 2,000 IU daily*

delicious, but if not, before taking a second bite, ask yourself, how much more of this meal do you want to eat and why? And if something doesn't taste great, don't eat it. You don't have to clean your plate. (Despite what your parents may have told you about the starving children of the world, no one will perish if you don't finish everything in front of you.)

- *If you are eating with others, talk about the food you are enjoying—how it looks, how it smells, and how it tastes. One of the joys of eating with my French in-laws is that we*

Shellfish Paella with Cauliflower Rice
(page 190)

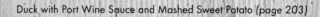
Duck with Port Wine Sauce and Mashed Sweet Potato (page 203)

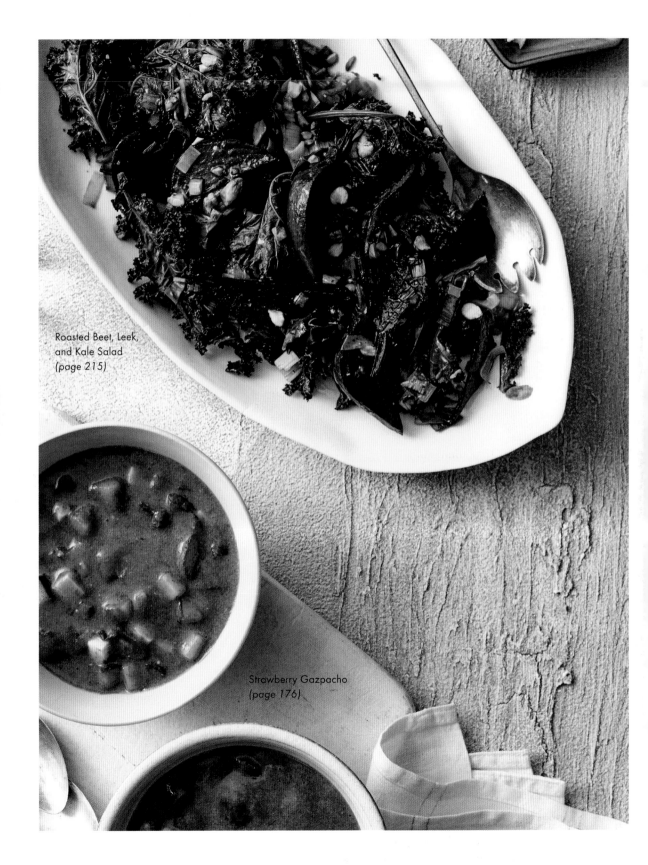

Roasted Beet, Leek,
and Kale Salad
(page 215)

Strawberry Gazpacho
(page 176)

Greek Lemon, Chicken, and Orzo Soup (page 177)
Greek Salad with Lemon Vinaigrette (page 183)

Marinated Mediterranean
Olives and Vegetables
(page 170)

Grilled Figs with
Port (page 223)

Arugula Salad with
Grilled Shrimp
and Fennel
(page 186)

Salade Niçoise (page 182), shown here served family style

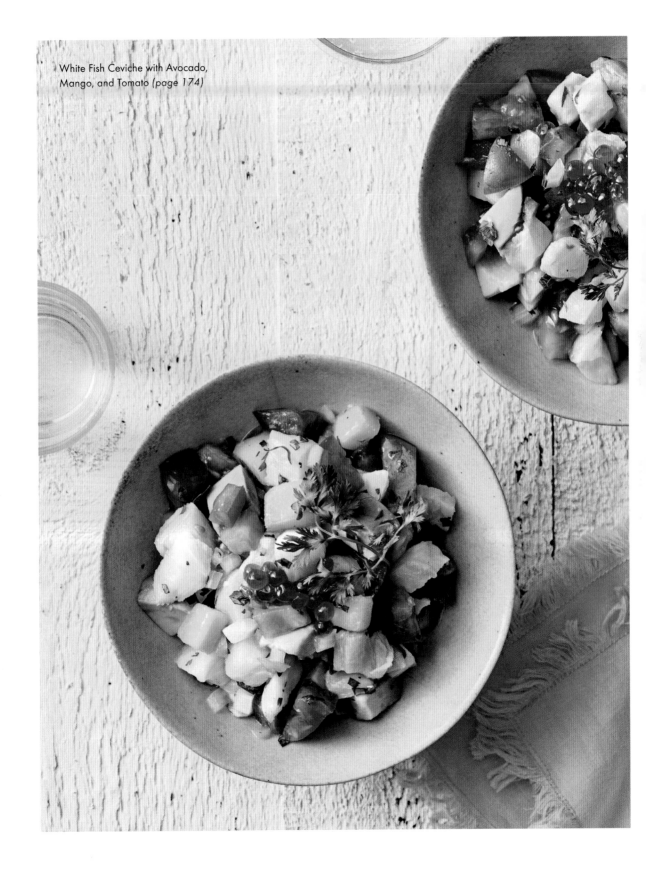

White Fish Ceviche with Avocado, Mango, and Tomato (page 174)

Berries and Yogurt with Toasted Muesli (page 165) and
Frittata with Spinach, Mushrooms, and Cheese (page 166)

Tzatziki (page 228) and
Method Hummus
(page 229)

Falafel Lettuce Wraps
(page 210)

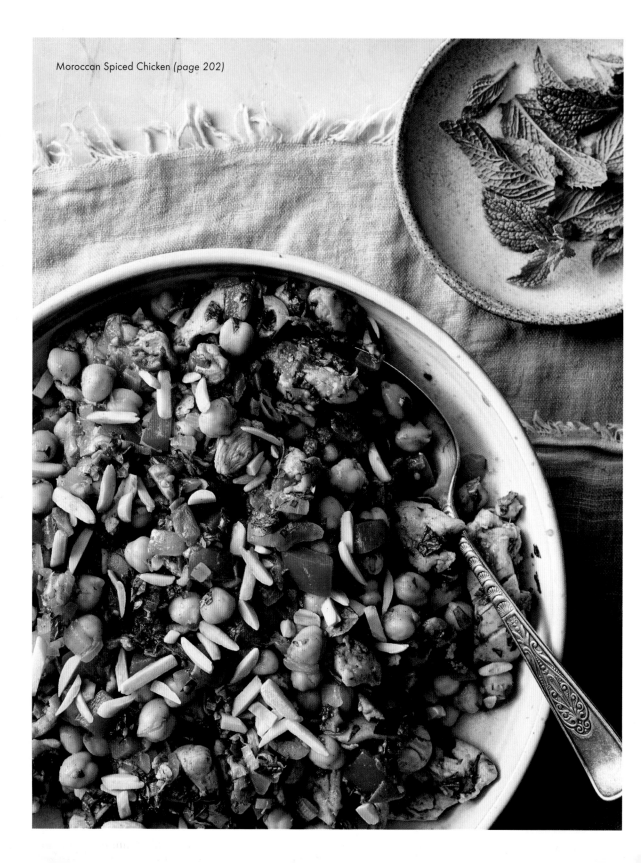

Moroccan Spiced Chicken (page 202)

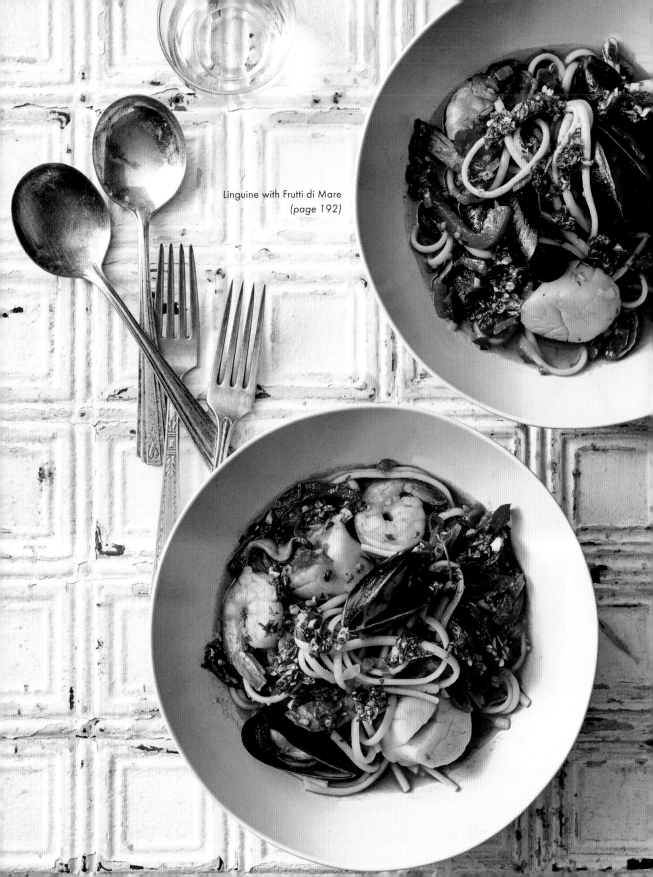

Linguine with Frutti di Mare
(page 192)

Mussels Marinière *(page 194)* and
Gigantes and Chard with Roasted Tomato,
Onion, and Garlic *(page 218)*

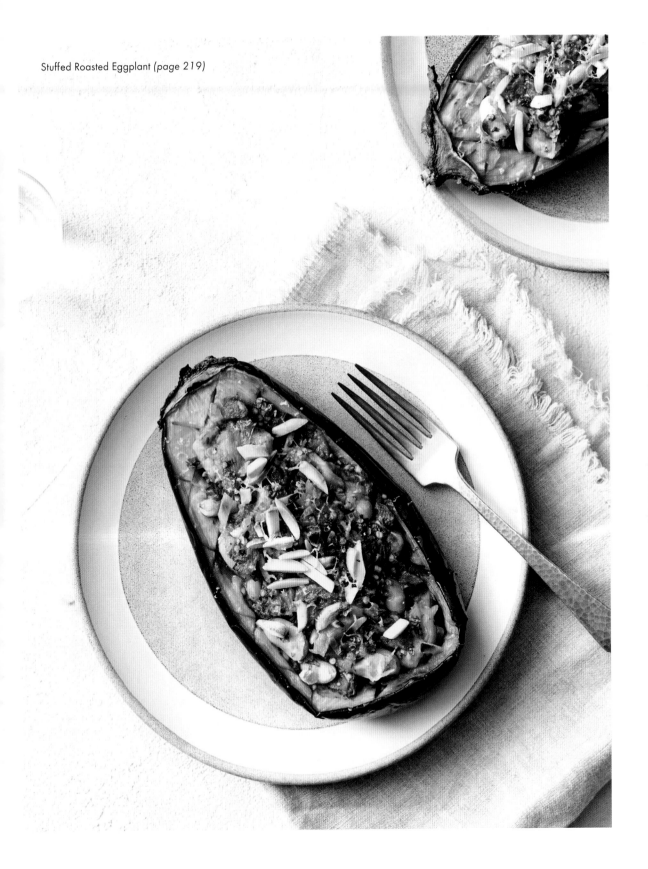

Stuffed Roasted Eggplant (page 219)

Chicken Breast with Pesto
and Mixed Greens (page 204)

Pears Poached with Wine
and Cinnamon (page 222)

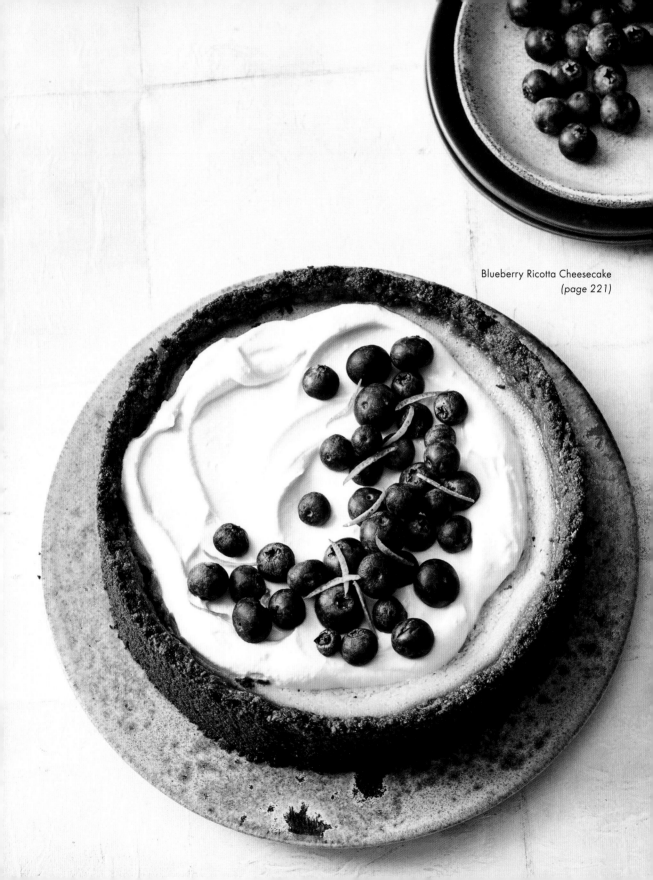

Blueberry Ricotta Cheesecake
(page 221)

always end up talking about what we are eating and drinking—which inevitably makes us appreciate our meal and our time together even more.

Probably the biggest challenge of mindful eating in our rushed world is that it calls for slowing down, not always easy given our jam-packed days. But it's so worth the extra time you will take to make your own food and set a place at the table for yourself (and, I hope, for others). If you practice mindful eating, very likely you will eat less, enjoy your food more, and make better choices.

TIMING IS EVERYTHING

For better blood sugar control, and especially if you are trying to lose weight, do as they do in the Mediterranean: Have a bigger lunch and a smaller dinner.

People in one study using a Mediterranean diet for weight loss lost more weight having 70 percent of their calories for breakfast, morning snack, and lunch, with only 30 percent of their calories for afternoon snack and dinner, compared to another group in the study who ate the exact same food, but with 55 percent of their calories in the morning and at lunch, and 45 percent in the late afternoon and evening. Over a twelve-week period, those eating more calories earlier in the day lost 18 pounds, compared to the bigger dinner group, who lost 13 pounds over the same twelve weeks. This suggests there is weight-loss benefit from eating a bigger lunch and a smaller dinner, which is often how food is consumed in Mediterranean countries. Those eating more earlier in the

day also showed greater improvements in insulin sensitivity. This supports prior studies showing that eating late at night, right before going to bed, decreases insulin sensitivity and promotes weight gain.

Even if you're not trying to lose weight and you're seeking to maintain your weight, it's clearly better for insulin sensitivity if you shift most of your calories to the first half of your day, rather than overdo it in the evenings. The worst thing to do is to eat within 60 to 90 minutes of going to bed.

RETHINK YOUR SNACK HABITS

Mediterranean people generally don't snack alone—if they snack at all—and when they do eat between meals, they do it very differently from how we often do it here. The idea of a person, all alone, eating ice cream out of the carton while standing at the kitchen sink, or eating a bag of potato chips in front of the TV, is a largely foreign concept in the Mediterranean. Indeed, eating alone isn't done by choice and snacking alone is unheard of.

Americans, on average, get 25 to 30 percent of their calories from snacking over the course of a day, which is nearly 600 extra calories, often from nutrient-deficient food. Southern Europeans in general don't snack, and my estimate is that at most snacking accounts for 10 percent of their calories.

Ironically, years ago when my French relatives visited us in the United States, they lost weight—but not by choice. That's because we offered healthy snacks such as hummus and sliced veggies, nuts, fruit, and yogurt while we were moving about and on the go, adding some calories in between moderately light lunches and dinners—meals that were smaller than what they were used to in France. (Back then my family snacked and ate low-fat meals, as we hadn't fully adopted a varied Mediterranean approach in our own home.) But they wouldn't snack on the go! They considered it taboo. Over the course of their visit they would take in fewer calories. The result was that they flew back home minus a few pounds.

For them and their countrymen (and women), eating is done (a) with others, and (b) at mealtime. Case in point: Aboard my boat in a Spanish port, I recently offered a local mechanic who was doing some repairs a quick taste of what I was cooking in the galley. He politely declined, saying that even though he was very hungry, it didn't seem right to just taste a bite while working, and he didn't have time to sit down for a meal!

That's not to say people never snack in the Mediterranean. It's just that when they do, it's often done with others while sitting at a table or in a living room with plates. For instance, before dinner out or at home with guests, there might be a drink—an aperitivo or apéritif—served with light fare. The idea is to take the edge off your hunger so that you don't devour your evening meal. Their light fare is generally healthier than American happy-hour food—instead of buffalo chicken wings with ranch dressing and unlimited appetizers, you'll find olives, nuts, stuffed grape leaves, vegetable sticks with hummus, maybe a small bit of thinly sliced cured meats, sardines—all depending on what part of the Mediterranean you're in. And—unless you're making a meal of small plates and Spanish-style tapas—these snacks are offered in very limited amounts because dinner is soon.

For some Mediterranean Method snack ideas, consider the appetizers and dips you'll find in Chapter 9, and make sure to keep staples like olives, nuts, and your favorite crunchy fresh vegetables on hand. Remember, it's too easy to tack on an extra 600 to 900-plus calories a day through snacking on nutrient-deficient foods. Snack mindfully!

MOVE YOUR BODY, REST YOUR MIND

You've gotten the message that exercise and daily activity are as important as choosing the right foods when following the Mediterranean Method. There are many ways to get active, and many structured exercise routines you can choose from. Pick something you enjoy, that fits your lifestyle, and that you'll stick with.

Add stress management to the mix, as well. You can eat the right foods and add the right mix of cardio and strength-training exercise, but if you ignore stress management, you won't get the benefits of a Mediterranean diet. Try meditation, yoga, or other mindfulness practices. You can also consider a program like HeartMath, an interactive software program that measures your state of calmness or agitation, and gives you feedback on how to relax, focus, and your ability to get calm. In my clinic, we measure your calmness or agitation level, much as your doctor might measure your blood pressure. It can be installed as a phone app or on your computer. I've found it to be a very effective tool to help people who are otherwise unable or unwilling to meditate and reduce their stress levels. See www.drmasley.com/resources for more information and a link to HeartMath.

Sufficient sleep is also important for lowering your risk of chronic disease and optimizing the power of the Mediterranean Method. Most adults need 7–9 hours of sleep per night—but many people try to get by on 6 hours, and it's not healthy, nor enough for optimal mental performance. If you're having serious trouble with sleep issues, see your physician. Here are a few quick tips if you are having some routine sleep challenges:

- *Watch what you're drinking.* Avoid drinking more than 2–3 servings of caffeine per day, and eliminate caffeine later in the day (especially if you're caffeine sensitive—see pages 39–40). Limit alcohol. Consuming more than a glass or two of any alcohol, including red wine, can cause a startle reflex, causing you to wake at around 2 a.m. In addition to keeping your intake moderate, avoid it within two hours before you go to bed.

- *Create a sleep-friendly environment.* Use your bedroom for sleeping, resting, and romance—not work and screen time. (I suggest getting the TV, the smartphone, and the computer out of your bedroom!) Keep your bedroom cool, use blackout shades and white noise machines if need be, and spring for a comfortable mattress, pillow, and bedding. Stress management can also help to promote sleep. People who regularly meditate have low levels of sleep deprivation—because they can fall asleep easily.

- *Be consistent.* Try to go to bed and wake up at the same times every day.

Dinner Out? Enjoy Small Plates—and Big Flavors

There is no reason to give up dining out with others if you follow a Mediterranean-style diet. On the contrary, sharing dinner out with others (or throwing a dinner party if you enjoy entertaining) works wonderfully with the Mediterranean Method. Inspired by the Spanish tradition of tapas, small-plate dining is a delicious and healthy option. Pick a restaurant that offers Mediterranean-style food, including plenty of vegetable dishes and seafood, and start by sharing a selection of appetizers. Or everyone can order his or her own individual soups or salads. Then move on to a few shared main courses, and order some extra vegetable side dishes. For dessert, select fresh fruit and cheese. Of course, the key is to pick the right restaurant—one that will be amenable to your "family-style" dining. Once you begin placing your orders, a welcoming restaurant will immediately see that you're not doing this to be "cheap"— and they'll accommodate you. (If not, leave—there are plenty of restaurants that would love your business!)

Hang On to These American Traditions

WHILE I'VE POINTED out a number of things we can improve upon in the United States—namely, the Standard American Diet and our lack of daily activity—there are a few important health-related habits that we get right on this side of the pond.

- *We don't smoke as much.*

Not smoking is one of the best habits on earth, for anyone. You'll up your chances of living without disease—including heart disease and cancer—and you'll live longer. Smoking cigarettes and cigars in Europe is far more prevalent than in this country. According to the CDC, 15.5 percent of Americans are smokers; in Europe, according to the European Commission, 26 percent of the European Union residents are smokers, with the heaviest concentrations in southern Europe, including Greece and France, where more than one-third of the population in each country smokes tobacco. (Note: These numbers don't account for the use of e-cigarettes/vaping.) While the United States has taken faster action to ban smoking from public spaces, including restaurants and bars, Europe has been much slower to take up such regulations. We are, without a doubt, more protected from secondhand smoke in this country. More than 700,000 E.U. residents die each year from tobacco-related deaths, but old habits die hard. I hope, if you smoke, that you can find the resources to quit.

- *When we eat breakfast, we eat protein.*

There is a growing trend in this country to include protein and avoid refined carbs for breakfast. Gone are the days when we encouraged dry cereal, pancakes, waffles, or toast. More people are shifting to having a protein shake for breakfast, or having eggs with vegetables, either scrambled or in a frittata or an omelet.

In Europe—not just in the Mediterranean—the morning meal gets short shrift. (Lunch, after all, is the big meal of the day.) It's either a quick espresso—or, for those who linger in a café, a cappuccino, café latte, or café con leche, café au lait . . . every country has a variation on a milky coffee drink for breakfast—and a few bites of bread or pastry, and maybe a bit of fruit. In other words, protein is rarely involved, but sugar often is.

But my advice to you is, *don't* do as the Europeans do: skip the morning sugar bomb and the idea of coffee and pastry (unless you're on holiday in a picture-perfect café). Having a sweet with breakfast or adding sugar to your morning coffee or tea is a particularly bad idea. That's because your cortisol levels naturally spike in the morning to wake you up, and physiologically make you less able to handle refined carbs. On the days you do have breakfast, make sure to have a protein boost such as yogurt, eggs, or a whole grain, such as steel-cut oats, with protein powder.

Protein in the morning is important—especially if you are trying to lose weight.

As mentioned in Chapter 3, to use the Mediterranean Method for weight loss aim for at least 20 grams of protein at breakfast. In a rush? See the recipe for Steven's Breakfast Shake on page 168—it delivers 20-plus grams of protein.

A Mediterranean Method Approach to Breakfast

Perhaps you first heard it from your mom: "Breakfast is the most important meal of the day!" For active, still-growing children and young people who have different needs than mature adults, generally a nutritious morning meal is quite important. But there are a lot of healthy people who don't like to eat breakfast for whatever reason, and they've been made to feel that it's an unhealthy habit—they'll overeat at lunch, they won't have any energy, and so on.

If you're healthy, I don't think it's a hard-and-fast rule that you always eat breakfast—it really does depend on how your body and brain feel in the morning. There are plenty of trim and fit Europeans who have only a quick espresso for breakfast, and don't eat until lunch (their most important meal of the day). Whether it's that quick espresso or a regular cup of black coffee or black tea (or maybe just water), that beverage-only approach is an idea I like to encourage, as it fits with the healthy trend of intermittent fasting (going 14–15 hours without eating, typically from 9 p.m. to noon, or 7 p.m. to 9 a.m.), growing in popularity among Americans and associated with improved weight loss and heart health (see pages 67–68), among other benefits. As part of the Mediterranean Method, experiment with skipping breakfast, at least a few days per week, and see how this lighter approach makes you feel. You can have black coffee or black tea, but don't add milk or sugar. You may like this new habit—it's very European.

Your Mediterranean Kitchen: Shopping and Cooking

ONE REASON WHY it's easy to follow a Mediterranean-style diet is that the ingredients are simple and fairly easy to find, and the cooking techniques themselves are quite basic. I love being in the kitchen and preparing food to share with friends and family, and things always go smoothly and quickly when I have the right items on hand. Here are some kitchen tools I find most valuable, followed by shopping guidelines for staples and fresh ingredients.

COOK'S TOOLS

Having the right tools makes cooking fun and easy. I live with two extremes. My home kitchen is loaded with gadgets and has a spacious pantry. In contrast, when I'm living on my sailboat with my wife, Nicole, the kitchen is very small and has limited storage space, so I have only the bare essentials, including:

KNIVES AND SCISSORS: Good chef's knives, my most important tools. I have both an 8-inch and a 12.5-inch blade, and a good paring knife, too, plus a couple pairs of kitchen scissors. I also have a knife-sharpening stone. (Ironic but true: You're much less likely to cut yourself with a sharp knife. Using a dull knife gets you in trouble every time.)

CUTTING BOARDS: At least two, one small and one large. Wood or plastic each has its advantages and both will work. Some people like glass, as it's easy to disinfect if you're cutting poultry, fish, or meat.

SAUTÉ PANS (OR SKILLETS): Small, medium, and large, preferably all the same shape so you can stack them to minimize storage space. Choose stainless-steel or anodized aluminum. Avoid pans made from cast iron, regular aluminum, or with Teflon or non-stick plastic linings.

SAUCEPANS: At least one small and one large, preferably stainless steel. On the boat I have three of them that stack to save space.

WOODEN SPOONS, SLOTTED SPOONS, SPATULAS, A WHISK: At least three wooden spoons. Different shapes and sizes come in handy, and when one gets dirty you'll always have a backup. I have a soft silicone spatula to scrape the side of a bowl, plus metal and plastic spatulas to flip or turn food in a pan. One medium-sized whisk is all you need.

BIG SOUP POT: Stainless steel. I like one that holds at least 8 quarts.

MESH STRAINER, COLANDER, SALAD SPINNER: I have all of them at home, but only a strainer and a colander when living on the boat.

MEASURING SPOONS, MEASURING CUPS: Choose glass measuring cups in 1-cup, 2-cup, and 4-cup sizes; I avoid plastic whenever possible in the kitchen, as chemicals will leak into your food.

PEELER, CHEESE GRATER, AND MICROPLANE FOR CITRUS ZEST: At home we also have a mandolin and a vegetable spiralizer, but on the boat I have only these three.

OVENPROOF BAKING DISHES: Glass or ceramic, preferably two, 9 by 13 inches.

BAKING SHEET WITH RIMS: Large size, great for roasting vegetables.

GLASS STORAGE CONTAINERS WITH PLASTIC LIDS: A variety of sizes that will stack to save space. Look for brands that can go from freezer to refrigerator to microwave or to the oven.

GLASS OR METAL MIXING BOWLS: Small, medium, large. Stackable stainless steel are the most practical.

MEAT THERMOMETER: Essential for cooking poultry, fish, or meat to the proper temperature.

BLENDER: Great for making smoothies and sauces. I also have a hand-held immersion blender for making small batches of sauces or puréeing.

FOOD PROCESSOR: Whatever size suits your needs. I have a few different sizes at home, but on the boat I use a 2-cup mini processor. Sometimes I have to work in batches to follow a recipe, but that's not a big problem.

Setting Up Your Pantry and Stocking Your Refrigerator

FROM DRIED INGREDIENTS and pantry staples to fresh produce and other fresh whole foods, keeping a supply of the right Mediterranean-themed ingredients makes all the difference when you're in the kitchen. Take a quick inventory and make sure your kitchen is taking on a Mediterranean flavor with these items.

HERBS AND SPICES

Stocking a good selection of dried herbs and spices, as well as having some fresh ones on hand, is a Mediterranean must. As you'll see

from my recipes, I like a variety of flavors (and therefore use a lot less salt as a seasoning). As for fresh herbs, you can easily grow most herbs in a small garden, in pots on a patio or balcony, and even on a windowsill. It's fun to do, and it's convenient and economical to have your own supply.

Dried Herbs and Spices

- Italian herb seasoning

- Fines herbes

- Thyme

- Oregano

- Sea salt

- Ground black pepper

- Dillweed

- Paprika

- Cayenne pepper

- Red pepper flakes (you can substitute cayenne if you generally don't use much spice)

- Curry spice blend

- Cinnamon

- Cardamom

Fresh Herbs

Grow your favorites! Here's what you'll probably use most:

- Parsley

- Mint

- Basil

- Rosemary

- Oregano

- Cilantro

- Garlic (you don't need to grow your own—but it's fun)

- Ginger (you can buy it fresh in most markets—cut off what you need and store the rest, unpeeled, in the refrigerator)

There are also perennial herbs such as chives, sage, and even lemon balm. Experiment with what you like to use for cooking or for making your own herbal teas and infusions.

OILS AND VINEGARS

- Extra-virgin olive oil (buy it in glass bottles, not plastic)

- Avocado oil (for cooking at medium-high heat or grilling)

- Almond oil (to have an alternative to avocado oil)

- Red wine vinegar

- Balsamic vinegar

- Optional: walnut oil for salads (a change from using only olive oil) and sherry or champagne vinegar for more variety

CONDIMENTS

- Hot sauce, gluten-free tamari sauce, salsa, Dijon mustard, vegetable broth, and/or chicken stock

CANNED OR JARRED STAPLES (CHOOSE BPA-FREE CANS)

- Beans: garbanzos (chickpeas), cannellini (white beans), and lentils. (You can also keep dried beans on hand if you want to soak them before using in recipes.)

- Artichoke hearts (packed in water or olive oil)

- Sardines (packed in olive oil)

- Olives (green, black, small, large)

- Tomato sauce and paste

NUTS AND SEEDS

Keep them in airtight jars in small quantities, or freeze big quantities and remove from the freezer to the pantry as you need them in small jars.

- Almonds (whole, slivered, and/or sliced)
- Pistachios
- Walnuts
- Pine nuts
- Sesame seeds

OTHER PANTRY ESSENTIALS

- Dark chocolate (preferably with at least 74% cacao)
- Protein powder (for shakes or to sprinkle on oatmeal—either grass-fed whey protein, or if you are dairy-free a pea/rice source of protein)

DAIRY (OR DAIRY-FREE SUBSTITUTES)

- Plain yogurt (Greek and/or regular), without added sugar or artificial sweeteners. (If you are dairy-free, look for nondairy yogurt options.)
- Parmesan or Parmigiano-Reggiano cheese for grating
- Organic, cage-free eggs
- Almond milk

FROZEN ITEMS

If you keep a well-stocked freezer, you'll never be out of meal options. Here's what I suggest you always have on hand:

- Poultry (look for organic, cage-free options): chicken and turkey breasts and thighs
- Fish (make sure they are individually packed and vacuum sealed or don't buy them frozen): Best is to always buy your fish fresh, but depending upon where you live that may or may not be realistic.
- Frozen berries

FRESH PRODUCE

Once you start using the recipes in this book, you'll get a good feel for what to keep on hand. Here are my favorites:

- Organic lemons and oranges (organic as you'll grate the peel into zest)
- Onions, garlic, shallots
- Avocados
- Green leafy vegetables (Plan to serve at least 1–2 cups per person every day with options such as kale, spinach, salad greens, chard, broccoli, etc.)
- Other vegetables (bell peppers, artichokes, tomatoes, fennel, green beans, celery, carrots, beets, butternut squash
- Fruit (berries, cherries, apples, pears, peaches, oranges—focus on whatever is in season)

Glycemic-Load (GL) Tables

MY MEDITERRANEAN METHOD emphasizes low-glycemic-load foods, as you know. Here are some listings for common foods, including many of the Mediterranean staples discussed in this book. This is how they're scored into low, medium, or high categories:

- 1–9 = Low GL
- 10–19 = Medium GL
- 20+ = High GL

Aim for low- and medium-GL foods and avoid high-GL choices—easy to do when you follow the Mediterranean Method!

FOOD OR BEVERAGE	AVERAGE SERVING SIZE	GLYCEMIC LOAD (PER SERVING)
BAKERY ITEMS		
MEDIUM GL		
Corn tortilla	50 grams (2 tortillas)	12
Pumpernickel bread	2 slices	13
Flour tortilla	50 grams (1 tortilla)	15
Rice cakes	1 ounce	18
Hamburger bun	2 slices	18
Cupcake, strawberry icing	1 cupcake	19
HIGH GL		
Whole wheat bread	2 slices	20
Wonder bread	2 slices (2 ounces)	20
Donut, glazed	One 4-inch diameter	22
Chocolate cake with icing	$\frac{1}{6}$th cake, 84 gm	25
Bagel, white	3.5-inch bagel	34
Baguette	3-inch piece	35

FOOD OR BEVERAGE	AVERAGE SERVING SIZE	GLYCEMIC LOAD (PER SERVING)
BEVERAGES		
LOW GL		
Unsweetened tea & coffee	1 cup	0
Almond milk (unsweetened)	1 cup	2.5
Skim milk	1 cup	9
Whole milk	1 cup	9
Soy milk	1 cup	9
MEDIUM GL		
Apple juice (unsweetened)	1 cup	12
Gatorade	1 cup	12
Orange juice (unsweetened)	1 cup	12
HIGH GL		
Cranberry juice cocktail (Ocean Spray)	1 cup	24
Coca-Cola	12-ounce can	25
Fanta (orange soda)	12-ounce can	35
CEREALS		
LOW GL		
Steel-cut oatmeal	1 cup	9
MEDIUM GL		
Oatmeal, rolled	1 cup	13
Cheerios	1 cup	13
Grits, cooked	1 cup	14
Special K	1 cup	14
Instant oatmeal	1 cup	16
All-Bran Cereal (Kellogg)	1 cup	16
Grape-Nuts	1 cup	16
Muesli (oats, nuts, dried fruit)	1 cup	16
Kashi Go Lean Crunch	1 cup	17

FOOD OR BEVERAGE	AVERAGE SERVING SIZE	GLYCEMIC LOAD (PER SERVING)
CEREALS		
HIGH GL		
Corn Flakes	1 cup	24
Raisin Bran (Kellogg's)	1 cup	26
Granola (Kashi)	1 cup	37
GRAINS		
MEDIUM GL		
Pearled barley (cooked, has gluten)	1 cup	11
Protein-enriched pasta (cooked)	1 cup	12.8
Spaghetti, whole-grain, boiled	1 cup	15
Bulgur wheat (cooked, has gluten)	1 cup	15.6
Wild rice, cooked	1 cup	16
Farro, cooked	1 cup	18
Quinoa, cooked	1 cup	18
Penne pasta (cooked)	1 cup	19
HIGH GL		
Brown rice, medium grain, cooked	1 cup	21
Sweet corn	1 cup	22
Spaghetti, white, boiled, 10 min	1 cup	22
Polenta (cooked)	1 cup	22.5
White rice, long-grain, cooked	1 cup	27
Quick-cooking white basmati	1 cup	28
Couscous, boiled 5 minutes	1 cup	30
Macaroni and Cheese (Kraft)	1 cup	32

FOOD OR BEVERAGE	AVERAGE SERVING SIZE	GLYCEMIC LOAD (PER SERVING)
COOKIES, SNACKS, CRACKERS, CHIPS		
LOW GL		
Hummus (chickpea salad dip)	30 grams	0
Guacamole	¼ cup	0
Dark chocolate (70–85% cocoa)	1 ounce	4
MEDIUM GL		
Popcorn, cooked	2 cups	12
Ginger snap cookies	1 ounce	17
Oatmeal cookies	1.5 ounces	18
Granola bar	2-ounce bar	18
HIGH GL		
Mars Bar	2-ounce bar	27
Potato chips	4-ounce bag	30
Pretzels, oven-baked	2-ounce bag	33
Tortilla chips, salted	3-ounce bag	35
DAIRY		
LOW GL		
Kefir	1 cup	1.8
Greek yogurt	1 cup	2.8
Milk (skim or whole fat)	1 cup	4.7
MEDIUM GL		
Low-fat yogurt with fruit, no sugar	1 cup	14
HIGH GL		
Ice cream, regular	1 cup	20 to 24
FRUITS		
LOW GL		
Apple	1 medium	6
Apricot	1 cup	6

FOOD OR BEVERAGE	AVERAGE SERVING SIZE	GLYCEMIC LOAD (PER SERVING)
FRUITS		
LOW GL		
Blueberry, wild	1 cup	1
Blueberry, commercially raised	1 cup	4
Cherries	1 cup	4
Grapefruit	1 small	3
Grapes	1 cup (120 grams)	5
Mango	1 cup (120 grams)	8
Orange	1 medium	4
Peach	1 large	5
Pear	1 medium	5
Pineapple	1 cup	7
Plums	1 cup	5
Strawberry	1 cup	3
Watermelon	1 cup	4
MEDIUM GL		
Apricot, dried	¼ cup	10
Banana, regular	1 medium	10
Banana, ripe	1 medium	16
Dates, dried	¼ cup	14
Fruit juice	1 cup	12
Papaya	1 cup	10
Prunes, dried	¼ cup	14
Raisins	¼ cup	18

FOOD OR BEVERAGE	AVERAGE SERVING SIZE	GLYCEMIC LOAD (PER SERVING)
BEANS AND LEGUMES		
LOW GL		
Black beans	½ cup	7
Chickpeas	½ cup	8
Navy beans	½ cup	7
Kidney beans	½ cup	7
Lentils	½ cup	6
Soy beans (edamame)	½ cup	3
White beans	½ cup	9
Peanuts	½ cup	1.7
Peas	½ cup	2.5
MEDIUM GL		
Baked beans	½ cup	10
HEALTHY FATS		
LOW GL		
Avocado	½ fruit	0
Olive oil, avocado oil, almond oil	1 tablespoon	0
Olives	1 ounce	0
Almonds	1 ounce	0
Hazelnut	1 ounce	0
Macadamia nut	1 ounce	0
Pecans	1 ounce	0
Pistachios	1 ounce	0
Walnuts	1 ounce	0
Peanuts (actually a legume)	1 ounce	0
Cashews, salted	1 ounce	3
Sunflower Seeds	1 ounce	7

FOOD OR BEVERAGE	AVERAGE SERVING SIZE	GLYCEMIC LOAD (PER SERVING)
VEGETABLES		
LOW GL		
Artichoke (Jerusalem)	1 cup	0
Asparagus	1 cup	3
Avocado	1 cup	0
Beets	1 cup	6
Bell pepper, green	1 cup	2
Bell pepper, red or yellow	1 cup	3
Bok choy	1 cup	0
Broccoli	1 cup	0
Cabbage	1 cup	0
Carrots	1 cup	2
Cauliflower	1 cup	0
Celery	1 cup	0
Fennel	1 cup	2
Mixed greens, lettuce, & raw spinach	1 cup	0
Parsnip	1 cup	8
MEDIUM GL		
Sweet potato, baked	1 medium (½ cup)	10
Potato salad	1 cup	13
Boiled white and purple potato	1 cup	14
Mashed potato	1 cup	17
HIGH GL		
Baked russet potato, average	1 medium (5 ounces)	26

FOOD OR BEVERAGE	AVERAGE SERVING SIZE	GLYCEMIC LOAD (PER SERVING)
LAND-ANIMAL PROTEIN		
LOW GL		
Steak, chicken, pork	6 ounces	0
Fish, shellfish	5 ounces	0
Eggs	2 eggs	0
ALCOHOL BEVERAGES		
LOW GL		
Red or white wine	5 ounces	0
Vodka	1.5 ounces	0
Beer (regular)	12 ounces	12.7
Light beer (6 grams of carbs/beer)	12 ounces	6
SWEETENERS		
Honey	1 tablespoon	10
Molasses	1 tablespoon	9
Maple syrup	1 tablespoon	8

Please Note: Various items may vary by a few points from one reference site to another.

9

MEDITERRANEAN METHOD RECIPES

BREAKFASTS

Mediterranean Wild Mushroom Omelet

A wild mushroom omelet provides a quick and easy way to prepare a fabulous meal. I grew up in the Pacific Northwest, and in the fall my family, led by my dad, would go gathering chanterelle mushrooms. Sometimes we'd make a mushroom omelet after we returned home—no matter the time of day. That's the beauty of an omelet: It can be breakfast, lunch, or dinner!

PREP TIME: 15–20 minutes | SERVES 2

4 tablespoons extra-virgin olive oil

8 ounces fresh wild mushrooms (such as cèpes, porcini, chanterelles, shiitakes, or oyster), trimmed and sliced

2 large shallots, minced

¼ teaspoon sea salt

¼ teaspoon ground black pepper

4 teaspoons water

1 cup chopped trimmed fresh kale

5 cage-free, organic eggs

½ cup grated Gruyère cheese (approximately 1½ ounces; see Note)

2 tablespoons chopped Italian flat-leaf parsley

Heat a large sauté pan or skillet to medium. Add 2 tablespoons of olive oil, then the mushrooms, shallots, salt, and black pepper, and sauté with an occasional stir until mushrooms and shallots have softened, about 2 minutes. Add 2 teaspoons of the water, stir the bottom of the pan, and add the kale; heat with a few stirs until it has wilted, another 2 to 3 minutes. Remove from the heat and cover.

Beat the eggs with the remaining 2 teaspoons of water in a small bowl.

To cook the eggs, you can use either the same large sauté pan (once you've cleaned the pan) and make a single large omelet, or for a technically easier method, use a medium pan and make two smaller omelets. The steps for making the omelet are basically the same.

Assuming you are making two smaller omelets for two people, heat a medium sauté pan over medium heat. Add 1 tablespoon of the olive oil, then pour in half the beaten egg mixture. After 1 minute, lift the edges of the egg, tilt the pan, let any uncooked egg flow under the cooked egg, and continue around the circle a couple times until egg is almost fully cooked and the bottom is golden, 2 to 4 minutes. Spoon half the cheese and half the mushroom mixture down the center of the omelet. Reduce the heat to low, fold one-third of each side of the omelet over the filling, and heat another 1 to 2 minutes.

Use a spatula to free the bottom of the omelet from the pan. Next, lay a plate over the omelet pan and invert the sauté pan, dropping the omelet onto a serving plate. Repeat these steps with the second omelet. Garnish the plates with parsley and, optionally, a couple tablespoons of remaining grated cheese. Serve immediately.

NOTE: If you are dairy-free, substitute 2 tablespoons of toasted slivered almonds for the cheese.

Berries and Yogurt with Toasted Muesli

This recipe yields two servings, which is perfect for my wife and me when we are at sea and need something filling, flavorful, and quick to pull together. We typically make a double or triple batch of muesli (toasted nuts, coconut, rolled oats, and cinnamon) so that we have enough for 4 to 6 servings; we store the extra in an airtight container for up to two to three weeks. You can substitute any nuts you have and use whatever fruit is in season.

PREP TIME: 10–12 minutes (2 minutes, with toasted muesli) | SERVES 2

½ cup old-fashioned rolled oats

1 tablespoon ghee (clarified butter)

¼ cup slivered almonds

¼ cup chopped walnuts

¼ cup unsweetened dried coconut flakes

¼ teaspoon ground cinnamon, or to taste

Pinch of sea salt

2 cups fresh berries

1 cup organic low-fat yogurt

Heat a skillet to medium-low, add the oats, and toast, stirring occasionally, until the oats are lightly browned, 3 to 4 minutes. Add the butter and stir to combine, then add the almonds, walnuts, coconut, cinnamon, and salt. Toast, with an occasional stir, for another 3 to 4 minutes. Remove from the heat.

When ready to serve, combine the berries and yogurt in a bowl, then mix in the muesli.

Frittata with Spinach, Mushrooms, and Cheese

The Italian equivalent of a crustless quiche, frittatas are simple to prepare and highly versatile—eat one for breakfast or prepare it as an entrée. Almost any vegetable will work—use what's in season. If you are dairy-free, use the spinach, onion, and mushrooms and turn this into an omelet without cheese.

PREP TIME: 20 minutes | BAKING TIME: 25 minutes | SERVES 4

8 ounces fresh spinach, washed, stems removed, leaves chopped

2 tablespoons extra-virgin olive oil, plus a little for the pie pan

½ medium sweet onion, finely chopped

2 cups sliced button mushrooms

½ teaspoon sea salt

2 garlic cloves, finely chopped

1 teaspoon Italian herb seasoning

8 large cage-free, organic eggs

2 tablespoons organic whole milk (or sour cream)

½ cup grated organic Conté (or Gruyère) cheese

¼ cup grated Parmigiano Reggiano cheese

Preheat the oven to 375°F.

Place the spinach in a saucepan with ½ cup water. Cover with a lid and allow to steam over high heat for 5 minutes. Remove from the heat and drain, squeezing out excess water.

Heat a sauté pan to medium hot, add the olive oil, and then the onion, and cook, stirring briefly; after 1 minute, add the mushrooms and continue cooking for 3 to 4 minutes, until the onion is translucent and the mushrooms have softened. Add the salt, garlic and herbs, and heat 1 minute more, then remove from heat.

In a large bowl, whisk together the eggs and milk, then add the cheese, spinach, and onion-mushroom mixture.

Grease a pie pan with a bit of the olive oil, then pour in the egg and vegetable mixture. Sprinkle the Parmigiano Reggiano cheese over the top. Bake for 25 to 30 minutes, or until it has the texture of custard—trembling and barely set in the middle. (If you'd like the top crust golden, place in the broiler for the last couple minutes of baking, but don't overbake, or it will be tough.)

Hot Steel-Cut Oatmeal with Apple, Berries, and Nuts

This recipe makes a hearty and nutrient-rich breakfast, especially nice on a cold morning. It also has a low glycemic load, so if you're a regular cereal eater, it's your best option. Nearly all other cereals have a higher sugar load. The optional extra protein will help rev your metabolism and keep you satisfied for half a day—just be sure to use grass-fed whey protein, or pick a rice/pea vegan protein powder option.

PREP TIME: 5 minutes, plus 30 minutes to simmer | **SERVES 2**

1¾ cups water

½ cup steel-cut oats

¼ teaspoon ground cinnamon

Pinch of salt (about ⅛ teaspoon)

1 medium apple, seeded, cored, and diced into ½-inch cubes

¼ to ¾ cup almond milk or organic low-fat milk

½ scoop vanilla or plain protein powder (optional; about 10 grams)

1 cup fresh berries

4 tablespoons chopped pecans (or other nut)

Place the water in a saucepan and bring to a boil. Add the oats, cinnamon, and salt, then reduce the heat and simmer for 10 minutes.

Add the apple, and continue to simmer for 10 to 20 minutes more, until the oats are tender. Just before serving, add milk as desired, and protein powder, if using. Serve in bowls with the berries and nuts scattered over the top.

Steven's Breakfast Shake

Shakes and smoothies aren't typical Mediterranean menu items, but since this one uses key Mediterranean ingredients, is loaded with heart- and brain-supporting nutrients, and provides clean protein to rev up the metabolism, I consider it a great option. As a bonus, it takes only 2 to 3 minutes to prepare!

PREP TIME: 2–3 minutes | SERVES 1

1 serving scoop (20 grams) protein powder (see Note)

½ cup frozen dark sweet cherries

1 large handful fresh or frozen baby kale leaves

1 tablespoon ground flax seeds (or chia seeds)

About 1 cup almond milk

Combine all the ingredients in a blender and purée until smooth. Pour into a glass. (Rinse the container immediately after to make cleanup easier.)

NOTE: If you need help finding a sugar-free, clean source of protein powder, visit www.drmasley .com/resources; I prefer whey protein for its immune-boosting properties and creamy texture, but if you are dairy intolerant, then select a dairy-free protein option instead.

APPETIZERS

Marinated Mediterranean Olives and Vegetables

In the markets all around the Mediterranean, vendors turn their unique combinations of olives, peppers, pickles, artichoke hearts, vinegar, and herbs into appetizer dishes—and often let you try their concoctions before you buy some. Use this recipe as a base from which to concoct your own favorite combinations. You don't have to use all the vegetables I list here, but try to use at least four of the six so as to have a variety of tastes and textures. If you prefer your olives pitted, then pit them just before mixing up this appetizer. I find that that pre-pitted olives are usually mushy and lack delicate flavors.

MAKES 2½ cups

DRESSING

1 tablespoon extra-virgin olive oil

1 tablespoon sherry vinegar or red wine vinegar

Zest and juice of ½ organic lemon

¼ teaspoon dried oregano

¼ teaspoon finely chopped fresh rosemary leaves

1 teaspoon honey

½ cup unpitted Kalamata olives, drained

½ cup unpitted green olives, drained

12 pepperoncini in vinegar, drained

⅓ cup extra-small dill pickles, drained

⅓ cup baby white onions in vinegar, drained

⅓ cup quartered jarred artichoke hearts, drained

In a small bowl, whisk the dressing ingredients together.

Combine the olives, pepperoncini, pickles, onions, and artichoke hearts in a bowl and toss with the dressing.

Refrigerate until serving, and serve with toothpicks.

Roasted Garbanzo Beans

Garbanzo beans are a good source of protein and fiber, and are surprisingly filling. When roasted like this, they also have a satisfying crunch. With the added herbs and spices, this easy-to-prepare appetizer is extra tasty.

PREP TIME: 10 minutes | ROASTING TIME: 30 minutes | MAKES 2 cups | SERVES 2-4

2 cups cooked garbanzo beans or 1 (15-ounce) can, rinsed and drained

2 tablespoons extra-virgin olive oil

¼ teaspoon sea salt

1 teaspoon paprika

⅛ teaspoon cayenne (optional)

½ teaspoon Italian herb seasoning

1 tablespoon finely chopped Italian flat-leaf parsley

Preheat the oven to 375°F.

Spread the beans on a rimmed baking sheet and roast for 10 minutes.

Meanwhile, in a small bowl, whisk together the olive oil, salt, paprika, cayenne if using, and herb seasoning. Add to the beans and stir to coat with the oil and spices, then return the beans to the oven, and roast another 20 minutes.

Transfer the beans to a serving bowl and garnish with parsley.

Spaghetti with Marinara Sauce and Mushrooms

I know what you're thinking: spaghetti in the appetizer section? Indeed, this is not a mistake!

In North America, we tend to serve spaghetti with sauce as a massive main course. In Italy, pasta comes before the main course of protein and vegetables, and the serving fits a small salad plate—enough for 8 to 10 wonderful bites—providing wonderful flavor yet a reasonable glycemic (sugar) load. There are endless possible variations, including adding roasted peppers, artichoke hearts, olives, and/or your other favorite vegetables. If you want to have a meat sauce, consider adding 1 pound of ground organic turkey breast or ground grass-fed sirloin to this recipe.

PREP TIME: 20–25 minutes

SAUCE COOKING TIME: 40–60 minutes (or several hours)

PASTA COOKING TIME: 8–10 minutes

MAKES 6 cups; SERVES 4 (with 1 cup sauce)

MARINARA SAUCE

4 tablespoons extra-virgin olive oil

1 medium onion, finely chopped

½ teaspoon sea salt

¼ teaspoon ground black pepper

1 tablespoon Italian herb seasoning

2 cups finely chopped button mushrooms

2 fresh medium tomatoes, finely chopped

6 medium garlic cloves, minced

2 tablespoons chopped fresh basil

½ cup dry red wine

1 (6-ounce) can tomato paste

1 (14-ounce) can tomato purée or tomato sauce

2 large dried bay leaves

Sea salt

2 to 3 ounces fiber- and protein-enriched spaghetti pasta

4 tablespoons grated Parmesan cheese (optional)

Make the sauce: Heat a large saucepan over medium heat. Add the olive oil, then the onion, salt, pepper, and Italian herbs, and sauté for 3 minutes, stirring occasionally. Add the mushrooms and cook another 3 minutes. Reduce the heat to medium, and add the tomatoes, garlic, and basil, and stir. Pour in the wine, and stir to free up any cooked bits at the bottom of the pan. Add the tomato paste and purée. When mixture begins to bubble, reduce the heat to a simmer, add the bay leaves, and simmer, covered, 40 to 60 minutes (or even several hours), stirring occasionally. Remove the bay leaves just before serving. (See Note.)

When ready to serve, heat a pot with about 2 quarts of salted water until water is briskly boiling. Add the pasta and stir initially to separate the spaghetti strands, then continue to stir occasionally while the pasta cooks. After 8 to 10 minutes, the pasta should be al dente (don't overcook); test for doneness and pour into a strainer.

While pasta is cooking, warm marinara sauce if not already heated.

To serve, add pasta to each plate, then add ½ cup of marinara sauce, stir minimally with pasta, then garnish with Parmesan cheese, if desired.

NOTE: This marinara sauce stores nicely—for up to a month in the freezer if you use an airtight container, or for several days in the refrigerator— so I typically make a large batch and store it in an airtight container.

White Fish Ceviche with Avocado, Mango, and Tomato

Around the Mediterranean, you'll see ceviche served everywhere, signifying that the fish has been "cooked" with citrus instead of heat. This is different from "à la tartar," which means that the fish is served raw. Either way, though, you'll want to use very fresh fish in this recipe, and if contemplating eating this à la tartar, be sure to check with your medical provider that consuming raw seafood is a safe option for you.

PREP TIME: 20–25 minutes | MARINATING TIME (FOR CEVICHE): 2 hours | SERVES 2

8 ounces sea bass fillet (or snapper or other white fish; see Note), diced into ½-inch pieces

4 to 5 lemons, juiced (about ¾ cup juice)

¼ teaspoon sea salt

¼ teaspoon ground black pepper

Pinch of cayenne

½ Hass avocado, diced into ½-inch pieces

1 fresh medium tomato, diced into ½-inch pieces

½ small mango, diced into ½-inch pieces

¼ small onion, minced

2 tablespoons finely chopped fresh cilantro, plus sprigs for garnish

2 teaspoons fish eggs (caviar or fish roe) (optional)

In a medium bowl, combine the fish with all but 2 teaspoons of the lemon juice, adding enough juice to totally cover the fish. Stir lightly to ensure all parts of the fish are in contact with the lemon juice. Cover and refrigerate for about 2 hours. Make a cut into the fish to ascertain it is completely opaque.

Drain the fish well in a colander. Return to a bowl, discarding the lemon juice marinade. Mix the fish with the salt, pepper, and cayenne to taste, and then add the avocado, tomato, mango, onion, cilantro, and remaining 2 teaspoons lemon juice. If desired, stir in half the fish roe and save the other half for a garnish, along with a few sprigs of fresh cilantro.

NOTE: Many grocery stores now carry sushi-grade white fish or ahi tuna. Either of these options would be good in this recipe, but skip the mango if you decide to use ahi.

SOUPS

Strawberry Gazpacho

Classic gazpacho is tomato-based, and hails from southern Spain. That's certainly a Mediterranean Method option, but this variation is too special not to include in this book. I had a version of this dish for the first time with friends in a restaurant in Portugal. The evening was warm, which made the chill of the soup all that much more refreshing.

PREP TIME: 15 minutes | CHILLING TIME: 10 minutes or more | SERVES 4

1 pound fresh strawberries, hulled

1 pound fresh cherry tomatoes

¼ cup loosely packed fresh herbs (basil, parsley, mint, thyme)

¼ teaspoon sea salt

¼ cup port wine

1 tablespoon fresh lemon juice

1 medium cucumber, diced

½ cup fresh organic mozzarella cheese, in ½-inch balls or ½-inch cubes

1 tablespoon finely chopped fresh mint

In a blender, purée half the strawberries with the tomatoes, herbs, salt, wine, and lemon juice.

Dice the remaining strawberries into ¼-inch pieces. Place the chopped strawberries in a serving bowl, then add the cucumber along with the purée. Finally, stir in the mozzarella and mint. Refrigerate for 10 minutes, or all day. Serve chilled.

Greek Lemon, Chicken, and Orzo Soup

This is an awesomely flavored soup, and with a deliciously creamy texture it's so good that you really don't need to add rice or pasta as would be traditional. Still, to keep this true to the original recipe, I left in a small portion of orzo pasta. If you're gluten-sensitive, leave that out.

PREP TIME: 20 minutes | COOKING TIME: 20 minutes | SERVES 4

2 tablespoons extra-virgin olive oil

1 medium onion, finely chopped

4 cups low-sodium chicken broth

2 cups water

2 medium carrots, diced

2 medium celery stalks, diced

12 ounces skinless, boneless chicken breast, diced into bite-sized pieces

½ cup orzo pasta

4 green onions, trimmed and chopped

4 cage-free, organic large eggs

¼ cup fresh lemon juice

2 teaspoons grated lemon zest

1 tablespoon finely chopped fresh dill or parsley

Heat a large pot to medium hot, then add the olive oil and onion and cook over medium heat until the onion is translucent, about 3 minutes. Add the broth and water, bring to a gentle boil, then add the carrots, celery, and chicken. Reduce the heat to medium-low and simmer for 10 minutes. Raise the heat to bring the liquid to a gentle boil again and add orzo. Reduce the heat to medium-low, add the green onions, and simmer for 7 to 8 minutes, until orzo is al dente. Remove from the heat when the orzo is cooked. *(This is not a soup that improves with longer simmering; total cooking time for the chicken should not exceed 10 minutes, or it might become tough; the orzo likewise should not be heated more than 8 minutes or it will be soggy.)*

Meanwhile, whisk the eggs until frothy in a large bowl. Add the lemon juice in a steady stream while continuing to whisk (it helps to have an assistant for this step, or just add a little at a time and whisk between additions). Still whisking, add 1½ cups of the hot broth to the eggs and lemon juice; the goal is a smooth creamy mixture without curdling the eggs.

When ready to serve, combine the egg-lemon mixture into the soup, stir in the lemon zest and dill, and serve at once.

Spanish White Bean Soup

Large white beans called fava beans (also called faba beans) are popular throughout the Mediterranean region, especially in Spain. If you can't find favas, large white broad beans are your best option. You could even substitute large kidney beans, lima beans, or cannellini beans. The traditional recipe for this soup calls for bacon or chorizo, but I don't think you'll miss the meat if you skip it. For the express version, using canned beans, see the tip following the recipe.

BEAN SOAKING TIME: 10–12 hours | PREP TIME: 20 minutes |
COOKING TIME: 1½ to 2½ hours (depends on type of bean) | SERVES 6

2½ cups large dried white beans

4 tablespoons extra-virgin Spanish olive oil

2 medium white onions, chopped

½ teaspoon sea salt

¼ teaspoon ground black pepper

2 medium carrots, chopped

1 green bell pepper, cored, seeded, and chopped

2 dried bay leaves

1 tablespoon red wine vinegar

1 teaspoon paprika

⅛ teaspoon cayenne (optional)

1 teaspoon dried thyme

8 medium garlic cloves, minced

½ cup finely chopped fresh parsley

2 cups low-sodium vegetable broth

4 cups water

Place the dried beans in a large bowl and add enough water to cover by 2 inches. Soak overnight (preferably 10–12 hours); drain in the morning and refrigerate until ready to cook.

Heat a large pot over medium heat, then add the oil, then the onions, salt, and pepper, and sauté, stirring occasionally, for 2 to 3 minutes, or until the onions soften. Add the carrots, green pepper, bay leaves, vinegar, paprika, cayenne if using, and the thyme, and heat another 3 to 4 minutes, with an occasional stir. (If you are adding chorizo or bacon, add along with the carrots and green pepper.) Add the garlic and parsley, and heat another 1 to 2 minutes.

Add the soaked beans, the broth, and water. Bring to a gentle boil, then reduce the heat to low, cover, and simmer for 1½ to 2½ hours, until the beans have softened, but are still slightly al dente.

When ready to serve, discard the bay leaves and ladle into bowls.

COOK'S TIP: You could use canned or jarred beans, but I find them always a bit overcooked, lacking the proper texture and flavor. Ideally—and if you have the time—you would use dried beans, soak them overnight, rinse them in the morning, and cook them the following day (details follow).

For the express version (ready in 30 minutes), skip the instructions for soaking the beans, and begin by heating the oil and sautéing the onions. Add the broth and water, and simmer 10 minutes. Add 4 (15-ounce) cans of white beans, drained and rinsed, and simmer for 10 minutes. Remove the bay leaves and serve.

Greek Lentil Soup

Great for lunch or a dinner appetizer, this dish is easy to prepare and is packed with healthy nutrients. Without the vinegar garnish, it will store well—sealed—in the refrigerator. But be sure to add that garnish when you do eat—it adds a delightful tanginess.

LENTIL SOAKING TIME: 1–4 hours | PREP TIME: 20 minutes
COOKING TIME: 1–2 hours (depending on lentil soaking time) | SERVES 4–6

1½ cups brown lentils

2 cups low-sodium broth

2 tablespoons extra-virgin olive oil

1 medium onion, chopped

2 cups chopped fresh tomatoes,
or 1 (15-ounce) can diced tomatoes

2 medium carrots, chopped

2 medium celery stalks, chopped

6 garlic cloves, minced

1 teaspoon dried rosemary

1 teaspoon dried oregano

3 dried bay leaves

Red wine vinegar to taste

Place the lentils in a medium pot, add enough water to cover by 1 inch, and let soak for 1 to 2 hours, and up to overnight (the longer they soak, the quicker they cook).

When ready to cook, bring the lentils in the pot to a boil, then reduce the heat to a simmer. Add the broth. Simmer for 30 minutes, then start testing the lentils every 15 to 20 minutes for doneness.

Meanwhile, heat a sauté pan to medium hot, then add the oil, and then the onion. Cook for 2 to 3 minutes, stirring occasionally, until the onion begins to soften. Add the tomatoes, carrots and celery, and cook for another 2 minutes. Stir in the garlic, rosemary, oregano, and bay leaves. Heat for 1 minute, then remove from the heat.

When lentils are about al dente, add the sautéed vegetables to heat through and cook the lentils a bit longer, until softened but not overcooked.

Serve the soup in bowls, drizzling each bowl with 1 to 2 teaspoons of vinegar.

Method Minestrone

This is one of my favorite soups of the week, meaning I make a big portion and enjoy it for dinner the first night, and then for lunches during the rest of the week. It is loaded with flavor and packed with healthy ingredients.

PREP TIME: 30–35 minutes | SERVES 5-6

¼ cup extra-virgin olive oil

1 medium sweet onion, chopped

2 medium carrots, chopped

2 medium celery stalks, chopped

8 baby portobello or button mushrooms, sliced

1 medium zucchini, diced

¼ teaspoon sea salt

¼ teaspoon ground black pepper

2 teaspoons Italian herb seasoning

½ cauliflower, trimmed and cut into 1-inch florets

4 fresh medium plum tomatoes, chopped, or 1 (15-ounce) can diced tomatoes

4 medium garlic cloves, minced

3 cups low-sodium vegetable broth

2 cups water

⅛ to ¼ teaspoon red pepper flakes (optional)

2 ounces elbow or mini-shell pasta

1 (15-ounce) can cannellini beans, rinsed and drained

1 (15-ounce) can red kidney beans, rinsed and drained

¼ cup Italian flat-leaf parsley, chopped

8 fresh basil leaves, sliced into thin strips

Few sprigs of fresh parsley

Heat a large pot to medium hot, add the olive oil and onion, and sauté for 2 minutes, with an occasional stir. Add the carrots, celery, mushrooms, zucchini, salt, pepper, and Italian seasoning and continue to cook for 4 to 5 minutes, stirring occasionally until vegetables soften.

Add the cauliflower, tomatoes, and garlic, and heat another 3 minutes. Then add the broth and water. Bring to a gentle boil, and add the pasta, then reduce the heat to a simmer and cook for 10 minutes. Add the beans and simmer another 2 to 3 minutes. Add the chopped parsley and basil and remove from heat. By this point, the pasta should be al dente, but not overcooked (see Note).

Serve in bowls with a sprig of parsley as a garnish.

NOTE: When this soup is ready to serve, unless you are serving to a large group, you don't want the leftover portions in a big pot to stay hot and overcook. Add some ice cubes or frozen vegetables to drop the heat and prevent overdone vegetables and pasta.

SALADS

Salade Niçoise

This is a modification of one of our favorite lunches to order when we are in France. The ingredients I use are packed with brain-promoting nutrients. Potatoes are more traditional than fennel, yet I've chosen fennel here for its nutrient-rich properties and lower sugar profile. Roasted beets can also be used in place of fennel or green beans, and canned pink salmon substitutes for the traditional canned tuna. Use any type of olives and tomatoes you find handy. The dressing is wonderful and can be used with many other salads, as well.

PREP TIME: 30 minutes | CHILLING TIME: 1–2 hours | SERVES 4

SALAD

1 tablespoon extra-virgin olive oil

1 large fennel bulb (about 8 ounces), trimmed and quartered; or 8 ounces small red potatoes (see Note)

¼ teaspoon sea salt

8 ounces fresh green beans, trimmed

1 large Bibb or Boston lettuce, larger leaves pulled off and flattened slightly

1 (6-ounce) can skinless, boneless red or pink salmon, drained

16 fresh cherry tomatoes, sliced in half

4 cage-free, organic large eggs, hard-boiled, then peeled and quartered

1 tablespoon drained capers

¼ cup Niçoise olives, pitted (or any other olive)

4 anchovy fillets (optional)

LEMON VINAIGRETTE

½ cup extra-virgin olive oil

¼ cup fresh lemon juice

1 tablespoon Dijon mustard

1 medium garlic clove, minced

⅛ teaspoon sea salt

⅛ teaspoon ground black pepper

½ teaspoon fines herbs

¼ cup fresh parsley, finely chopped

Heat a sauté pan to medium hot, then add the oil, fennel, and salt. Sauté for about 5 minutes, turning occasionally, until fennel is lightly golden. (If using potatoes instead, see Note.)

In a large saucepan, blanch the green beans in boiling water for 90 seconds, or until al dente, then drain and add to ice water to arrest the cooking. Refrigerate the fennel and beans for at least 1 hour, to chill thoroughly.

Whisk the dressing ingredients together and let sit at room temperature.

When ready to serve, place the large lettuce leaves on large individual plates. In the center of each, make a mound of salmon. In a circle around it, create separate mounds of fennel quarters and tomato halves, then add some green beans and egg quarters. Garnish each plate with some capers, olives, and anchovies. Drizzle the dressing over each salad and serve.

NOTE: If using potatoes in lieu of fennel, bring a large pot of salted water to a boil. Add the potatoes and cook until tender but still firm, about 15 minutes. Drain and cool.

Greek Salad with Lemon Vinaigrette

In Greece, salad really isn't about lettuce—instead it's a bounty of other wonderful, local produce. If you want to turn your salad into a full meal, add two cups of cooked, drained, and rinsed garbanzo beans. Regarding olives, as I've said, pitted olives that come in a jar or can tend to be mushy and lose flavor, so it's far better to buy unpitted olives in a jar, and remove the pits just before serving.

PREP TIME: 20–25 minutes | SERVES 4

1 medium red onion, thinly sliced

4 fresh medium tomatoes, cut into bite-sized wedges

1 large cucumber, sliced

1 red bell pepper, cored, seeded, and chopped

1 green bell pepper, cored, seeded, and chopped

8 ounces Kalamata olives, drained and pits removed

4 tablespoons drained capers

¾ cup crumbled feta cheese (about 2 ounces)

DRESSING

8 tablespoons extra-virgin olive oil

1 lemon, juiced (3–4 tablespoons)

1 teaspoon dried oregano

¼ teaspoon freshly ground black pepper

In a large salad bowl, combine the onion, tomatoes, cucumber, bell peppers, olives, and capers.

Whisk the dressing ingredients together in a small bowl, then pour the dressing over the salad, toss well, then garnish with the feta and serve.

Tabbouleh

Tabbouleh is a simple preparation, but don't let its simplicity fool you—it is a deliciously filling and wonderful side dish, and it complements almost any form of protein to make a complete meal. If you are gluten sensitive, substitute quinoa for the bulgur wheat.

The cherry tomatoes add great color and flavor, but while tabbouleh will store well, the tomatoes won't, so add the tomatoes just before serving.

PREP TIME: 30 minutes | SERVES 4

½ cup fine bulgur wheat

1 cup boiling water

2 tablespoons fresh lemon juice

4 tablespoons extra-virgin olive oil

½ teaspoon sea salt

¼ teaspoon ground black pepper

1 cup Italian flat-leaf parsley, finely chopped

½ cup fresh mint, finely chopped

1 small cucumber, half-peeled in lengthwise strips, then cut into ½-inch pieces

4 green onions, trimmed and finely chopped

1 cup fresh cherry tomatoes, sliced into quarters

Place the bulgur in a medium bowl and pour in the boiling water. Cover and let stand 15 minutes (or follow package directions). Drain in a sieve, pressing on the bulgur to remove any excess liquid.

Transfer the bulgur to a serving bowl and mix in the lemon juice, olive oil, salt, and pepper. Then toss in the parsley, mint, cucumber, green onions, and tomatoes.

Cover and refrigerate at least 30 minutes prior to serving. (As noted, if refrigerating all day, add the green onions and tomatoes just prior to serving.)

Spanish Mixed Salad with Mustard Vinaigrette Dressing

This can be served as a light main course or as a side dish with more protein. There are dozens of variations on this popular Mediterranean salad. Typically, it comes with canned tuna, although I prefer a fish with less mercury and more omega-3 fats, so I use canned sardines or pink salmon instead. You can substitute any vegetables that are in season.

PREP TIME: 25 minutes | SERVES 2

VINAIGRETTE DRESSING

5 tablespoons extra-virgin olive oil

1½ tablespoons red wine vinegar

1 tablespoon dry white wine

¼ teaspoon Dijon mustard

1 medium garlic clove, diced

⅛ teaspoon sea salt

SALAD

4 cups mixed greens

2 cage-free, organic eggs, hard-boiled and sliced in half lengthwise (see Note)

1 cup julienned raw beet, parboiled

½ cup shredded raw carrot, parboiled

12 black and/or green unpitted olives

1 cup quartered jarred artichoke hearts

1 medium Hass avocado, pitted and sliced into quarters

½ orange or red bell pepper, cored, seeded, and julienned

8 fresh cherry tomatoes, sliced in half, or 2 medium tomatoes, sliced into wedges

1 (4- to 5-ounce) can sardines packed in olive oil (or pink salmon), drained

Whisk together the vinaigrette dressing ingredients in a small bowl.

In a large bowl, toss the greens with 3 tablespoons of the dressing and then spread the greens on 2 serving plates. Add half an egg to opposite sides of each plate, then create a circle of mounds of shredded beets and carrots, olives, artichoke hearts, avocado, bell pepper, and tomatoes. Add the sardines to the center. Finally, drizzle the remaining dressing over the vegetables and serve.

NOTE: To prepare hard-boiled eggs, gently place the eggs in a small saucepan and cover with water. Set pan over moderate-high heat and bring the water to a boil. Once boiling, turn off the heat and wait 8 minutes. Remove the eggs and allow to cool before peeling.

Arugula Salad with Grilled Shrimp and Fennel

This is a wonderful salad for lunch or dinner, easy to prepare and super flavorful. Arugula is sometimes called "rocket." The kind of shrimp you use matters here. Shrimp caught with trawlers effectively rake the bottom of the sea and are very destructive. By contrast, the Mediterranean Sea is dotted with shrimp pots, which is an environmentally-friendly way to harvest the shrimp. Even outside Europe, you can now often find pot-harvested wild shrimp in grocery stores or online. Wherever you get them, look for a "Sustainable Fisheries Partnership" logo to ensure they were collected in a sustainable way.

THAWING TIME: 10 minutes

PREP TIME: 20–25 minutes

MARINATING TIME: 10 minutes

SERVES 2

¾ pound fresh or frozen large shrimp in the shell, thawed (see Note)

3 tablespoons avocado oil

2 medium garlic cloves, minced

1 tablespoon fresh lemon juice

½ teaspoon sea salt

½ teaspoon paprika

1 medium to large fennel bulb, trimmed and outer layers discarded, bulb sliced lengthwise into ¾-inch wedges

3 tablespoons extra-virgin olive oil

1 orange, peeled with a knife and segments separated

2 tablespoons pine nuts, lightly toasted (or chopped pistachios or almonds)

4 cups arugula (rocket), trimmed

In a bowl, marinate the thawed shrimp in a mixture of the avocado oil, garlic, lemon juice, ¼ teaspoon salt, the paprika, and the fennel wedges for 10 minutes.

Preheat a grill or broiler to medium-high.

In a salad bowl, combine the olive oil and remaining ¼ teaspoon salt, then break open 1 or 2 orange segments and add 1½ tablespoons of juice. Whisk together.

With a slotted spoon, scoop out the shrimp and fennel from the marinade; discard the marinade.

First, grill the fennel slices for 3 to 4 minutes on one side. Turn and grill on the other side for another 3 to 4 minutes. While the second side is grilling, add the shrimp and grill for 2 to 3 minutes per side, until the shrimp are pink and curled, but not overcooked. Remove the fennel slices from the grill and place in the salad bowl. Then remove the shrimp and set aside.

Heat a small sauté pan to medium hot and toast the pine nuts for 1 to 2 minutes, until warm and fragrant, then set aside.

Place the arugula in the salad bowl and toss with the fennel and vinaigrette. Add the shrimp on top and garnish with the pine nuts. Serve immediately.

A NOTE ON SHRIMP: Much shrimp sold in markets is either fast-frozen raw or cooked and then frozen, either with or without the shell. If posted as "previously frozen," the shrimp may have been thawed several days ahead, during which time its flavor declined. Unless you can buy fresh shrimp in the shell that's never been frozen, it's best to buy the shrimp frozen for this recipe and thaw it yourself. And if you are lucky enough to find fresh whole shrimp (with the heads), you'll need to buy 1½ pounds for this recipe, then marinate and grill the shrimp with the heads and shells intact, and serve whole.

To thaw and prepare the frozen shrimp, soak them in a large bowl with tap water, then remove the shells, devein, and drain and pat dry with paper towels.

White Bean and Celery Salad

This is a popular chilled salad and easy to prepare, as you don't have to cook anything. It can be served as a first course, light meal, or side dish. You can substitute a variety of white beans, vegetables, and herbs as desired. It's best to soak the beans overnight, rinse, and then cook them until they are al dente but not overly soft. Home-cooked beans always have the best texture. Admittedly, I'm not always that organized, and canned beans make this salad quick and easy. The tomatoes won't store well, so only add them to portions you will serve in the next couple hours.

PREP TIME: 15 to 20 minutes (not including bean cooking time) | SERVES 2 for full mean, 4 as side dish

3 tablespoons extra-virgin olive oil

1 tablespoon red wine vinegar

½ teaspoon sea salt

¼ teaspoon ground black pepper

½ teaspoon dried thyme

2 medium garlic cloves, minced

2 (15-ounce) cans navy beans, rinsed and drained (or 2 cups home-cooked beans; see Note)

2 medium celery stalks, finely diced

¼ cup Italian flat-leaf parsley, finely chopped

1 cup fresh cherry tomatoes, sliced in half

In a salad bowl, whisk together the olive oil, vinegar, salt, black pepper, thyme, and garlic. Add the beans, celery, parsley, and tomatoes. Toss together and refrigerate for at least 30 minutes, but not more than 1 to 2 hours.

NOTE: If preparing your own beans, soak 1 cup dried navy beans overnight, then rinse and place in a pot with salted water to cover. Bring to a boil, then simmer for 30 to 60 minutes, or until al dente. Rinse beans in cold water and drain.

SEAFOOD DINNERS

Shellfish Paella with Cauliflower Rice

Paella is a staple in Spain, but the traditionally excessive amount of rice makes for an unhealthy glycemic load. I discovered that substituting cauliflower rice (cauliflower that has been finely chopped in a food processor) makes this dish easier, quicker to prepare, dramatically healthier, and equally delicious.

PREP TIME: 20 minutes | COOKING TIME: 20–25 minutes | SERVES 4

¼ cup vegetable broth (or fish broth or white wine)

2 pinches of saffron threads (¾ to 1 teaspoon; see Note)

¼ cup extra-virgin olive oil

1 medium sweet onion, finely chopped

¼ teaspoon sea salt

1 medium red bell pepper, cored, seeded, and diced

4 cups fresh or thawed frozen cauliflower rice

1 teaspoon paprika

1 teaspoon dried oregano

Grated zest of 1 medium organic lemon

4 medium garlic cloves, minced

2 fresh medium tomatoes, chopped

1 cup fresh or thawed frozen peas

1 pound large shrimp or prawns, peeled and deveined

1½ to 2 pounds littleneck clams and/or mussels in the shell

½ cup Italian flat-leaf parsley, chopped

In a saucepan, heat the broth until hot but not quite boiling. Pinch the saffron threads between your fingers to crush them. Add them to the broth, and allow them to soak for about 15 minutes.

Heat a large wide pan (I use a 16-inch paella pan, but you could use a large 16-inch skillet or two 8- or 9-inch sauté pans) to medium hot and add the olive oil, then add the onion and salt, and cook for 2 to 3 minutes, stirring intermittently until onion is translucent. Add the bell pepper and cauliflower rice, and cook another 2 minutes, stirring occasionally. Stir in the paprika, oregano, lemon zest, garlic, tomato, and heat for 3 more minutes. Reduce the heat to medium low, pour in the broth with the saffron, and simmer with an occasional stir for 5 minutes.

Sprinkle in the peas, then add the shrimp, clams, and/or mussels (with shells positioned on their hinges so they open facing up). Cover the pan with a lid or aluminum foil, and simmer for 12 to 14 minutes, or until the seafood is nearly cooked and clams and mussels have opened. Avoid stirring after adding the seafood, so that the vegetables can develop a little crunchiness. Uncover, and simmer another 5 minutes. Serve immediately, sprinkled with the parsley.

A NOTE ON PAELLA: The word "paella" comes from the phrase "para ella," which in Spanish means "for her." In the distant past in Spain, women and men ate separately. The men were served first, with generous portions of poultry, sausage, seafood, and rice, and the women basically ate together and got the leftovers. But when you sauté onions, vegetables, and rice, add whatever protein you have on hand—poultry, sausage, seafood, or all three—and then add a tiny bit of a precious spice, you aren't exactly getting second best! The result is one of Spain's most popular and delicious dishes.

The only challenge with this amazing dish is buying that precious spice: saffron.

It is expensive because the saffron crocus (*Crocus sativa*) is an extremely labor-intensive crop. Each flower has three tiny, threadlike stigmas in the center, and these are typically picked by hand. The result is an amazing, concentrated flavor. Saffron threads may be hard to find (though now it is easy to order online), and ¾ to 1 teaspoon (which is $^1/_{10}$ ounce) may cost anywhere from $5 to $10. If you can't get it, you can still enjoy this dish without the saffron, although I hope you'll find that the occasional treat in this amazing meal is totally worth it!

Linguine with Frutti di Mare

You'll notice that this dish has triple the vegetables and half the pasta of the traditional restaurant-cookbook portion, increasing the flavor and lowering the sugar load of this wonderful dish. When available, select fiber- and protein-rich pasta, such as Barilla brand; it has double the protein, double the fiber, and far less refined carbs. Choose the freshest shellfish available or use frozen options— if so thaw, drain, and pat dry—selecting the best mussels, shrimp, sea or bay scallops, clams, or squid available.

PREP TIME: 30–35 minutes | SERVES 4

⅓ cup extra-virgin olive oil

1 medium onion, finely chopped

2 teaspoons Italian herb seasoning

¼ teaspoon sea salt

¼ teaspoon ground black pepper

¼ to ½ teaspoon red pepper flakes

3 cups sliced button mushrooms

1 medium bell pepper, cored, seeded, and sliced

4 fresh medium tomatoes, chopped

8 medium garlic cloves, minced

1¼ cups Italian flat-leaf parsley, finely chopped

4 ounces linguine fiber- and protein-enriched pasta

¾ pound large shrimp, peeled and deveined

8 large sea scallops (about 8 ounces)

2 tablespoons avocado oil

¼ cup dry white wine

¾ pound mussels in the shell, rinsed and beards removed (or littleneck clams)

Bring a pot of salted water to a boil.

Meanwhile, heat a large sauté pan to medium hot, add 3 tablespoons of the olive oil, then add the onion, herbs, salt, pepper, red pepper flakes to taste, and mushrooms and cook, stirring occasionally, for 3 minutes. Add the bell pepper and tomatoes and continue to cook another 2 to 3 minutes, stirring occasionally. Add half of the garlic and half the parsley, then cook 2 minutes more, until the garlic is softened but not browned. Transfer to a large bowl and set aside.

When the water is boiling briskly, add the pasta, stirring occasionally, and cook for about 8 minutes or until the pasta is al dente, ideally slightly undercooked. Drain well, and add to the bowl with the vegetables.

While the pasta is cooking, pat dry the shrimp and scallops with paper towels.

Using the same sauté pan as earlier, heat it to medium-hot. Add the avocado oil, then the shrimp and scallops, and sear both for 30 seconds on each side. Pour in the wine, then add the mussels, cover the pan, and steam for 3 to 4 minutes, until the mussels open. Discard any mussels that don't open, then pour the vegetable-pasta mixture into the pan, stir to mix well, cover the pan, and heat for 1 to 2 minutes, until warmed through.

Bring a small sauté pan to medium hot, then add the remaining 3 tablespoons olive oil and the remaining parsley and garlic. Simmer over low heat for 2 minutes, until garlic is softened but not browned.

With tongs, transfer the pasta, shellfish, and vegetables to a serving platter. Drizzle the parsley sauce over and serve.

Mussels Marinière

Here is a classic French seafood dish that is easy to prepare and tastes fantastic. The key is finding fresh mussels—they should smell like the sea. The majority of mussels that you'll find in the store are farm raised, which is fine here, as wild or farm raised both feed off the same plankton. What is important is that the mussels are raised in clean water.

PREP TIME: 20-30 minutes | SERVES 4

4 to 5 pounds mussels in the shell

2 tablespoons organic butter

2 tablespoons extra-virgin olive oil

2 small onions, sliced

2 medium garlic cloves, minced

½ teaspoon herbes de Provence or Italian herb seasoning

½ cup Italian flat-leaf parsley, chopped

1 cup dry white wine

Scrub the mussels with a soap-free brush under cold running water. Pull off any beards (the brown tuft of fibers emerging from the shell). Discard any mussels that do not close when you tap them with your finger, as well as any with broken shells.

Heat a large pot to medium hot, then add the butter, olive oil, and onions, and sauté for 3 minutes, or until onions soften. Add the garlic, the herbes de Provence, and half the parsley and sauté another minute. Pour in the wine and stir to loosen the bits adhering to the pan bottom.

Bring the mixture to a boil, then lower the heat and cook 2 minutes. Add the mussels, and cover the pan. Stirring every 1 to 2 minutes, cook just until the shells open, 3 to 4 minutes. Remove the mussels from the sauce using a slotted spoon, and place in serving bowls.

Strain the cooking liquid and return it to the pot. Add the remaining parsley, stir, then drizzle over the mussels as a garnish.

Grilled Sea Bass

Sea bass is on most menus in the Mediterranean, and is often served with a simple olive oil, lemon, and herb sauce. You can substitute snapper for bass, if that's what looks good in the market that day. The key is to use *fresh* fish; whenever feasible, ask to smell the fish before they wrap it and decline it if it smells "fishy." I recommend serving this with grilled vegetables and/or a mixed salad.

PREP TIME: 15 minutes | GRILLING TIME: 15 minutes | SERVES 2

1 (1½-pound) whole sea bass, cleaned (see Note)

2 tablespoons avocado oil

½ teaspoon sea salt

½ teaspoon ground black pepper

SAUCE

4 tablespoons extra-virgin olive oil

2 tablespoons fresh lemon juice

1 tablespoon Italian herb seasoning

1 garlic clove, minced

Rinse the fish and pat dry. Lay flat on a work surface. From behind the head to the tail, make shallow cuts crosswise about ¼ inch deep down both sides of the fish every 1½ inches.

Preheat a grill or broiler.

Rub the avocado oil, salt, and pepper over the fish, inside and out. Place on the grill and cook for 6 to 8 minutes per side, until lightly browned. When the internal temperature reaches 150–155°F, remove from the grill and place on a serving platter.

Whisk the sauce ingredients together.

Remove the skin from the fish and carefully lift off the fillet pieces from the top, then flip the fish and repeat for other side. Place the fish pieces on plates, and drizzle the sauce over.

NOTE: Traditionally, sea bass is grilled with the head on and without removing the scales, keeping the flesh tender. Removing the head causes the fish to lose moisture when cooking; removing the scales makes the fish meat a bit drier on the grill. However, if you enjoy eating the skin (in truth the skin is loaded with nutrients and healthy fats), have the fishmonger remove the scales; if not, keep the scales on the fish and remove the skin after it has been grilled and before the fillets are plated. The only reason to remove the head is if your grill isn't big enough for the fish to fit.

Cioppino (Italian-Style Seafood Stew)

This is one of our favorite meals to serve when we have company. It makes an elegant presentation, steaming hot and exotic. Be sure you buy very fresh fish and shellfish, and vary your vegetables (and seafood) according to availability. This stew is great to serve with a tossed green salad as a second course.

PREP TIME: 20 minutes | SIMMERING TIME: 30 minutes | SERVES 4

1 tablespoon extra-virgin olive oil

1 medium onion, chopped

¼ teaspoon sea salt

1 cup sliced button mushrooms

1 teaspoon Italian herb seasoning

¼ teaspoon ground black pepper

3 large carrots, chopped

1 medium-large fennel bulb (or 3 celery stalks), trimmed and chopped into ½-inch pieces

1 cup dry red wine

1 medium red bell pepper, cored, seeded, and chopped

1 cup chopped fresh tomato or tomato sauce

2 cups low-sodium vegetable or fish broth

2 cups water

1 pound mussels and/or littleneck clams in the shell, scrubbed clean and any beards removed

1 pound white fish fillets (tilapia, cod, snapper, sea bass), cut into 1-inch pieces

8 ounces large shrimp, peeled and deveined (or stone crab legs in the shell)

8 sea scallops

½ cup Italian flat-leaf parsley, finely chopped

Heat a large pot over medium heat. Add the oil, then add the onion, salt, mushrooms, Italian herbs, and black pepper, and stir for 2 to 3 minutes. Add the carrots and fennel and cook another 2 minutes. Pour in the wine to deglaze the pan for 30 seconds, while stirring (the wine helps release the onion's sugars that are stuck to the pan). Add the bell pepper, tomato, and broth, bring to a gentle bowl, then reduce the heat and simmer for 15 to 20 minutes.

Meanwhile, pour the water into another pan fitted with a steamer tray and bring the water to a boil. Add the mussels and/or clams, and cook until they open, 5 to 6 minutes. Drain, saving 1 cup of the steaming liquid.

Increase the heat under the pot to medium-high and add the fish along with the shrimp and scallops. Cook for 4 to 5 minutes, until the shrimp are pink and the fish is opaque. Add the mussels and/or clams, plus the reserved steaming liquid, and simmer another minute.

To serve, ladle into bowls and garnish with the parsley. Be sure to set the table with a second batch of large bowls for discarded shells.

Baked Trout and Vegetables with Herbes de Provence

Trout, a freshwater fish, is popular in Spain, France, and Italy, and it holds up well, especially when baked whole. As with all fish, though, freshness is key. How can you be sure? The skin should glisten and the eyes should be shiny and plump. If using trout fillets instead, just reduce the cooking time to 10 to 12 minutes; you want the fillets to remain moist.

PREP TIME: 20 minutes | BAKING: 25 minutes | SERVES 2

4 tablespoons extra-virgin olive oil

1 medium red onion, thinly sliced

1 medium fennel bulb, trimmed and thinly sliced lengthwise

2 medium carrots, sliced

1 cup chopped zucchini (1 small)

¾ teaspoon sea salt

1 tablespoon plus 1 teaspoon herbes de Provence

1½ pounds whole trout (1 large or 2 small)

2 medium garlic cloves, minced

Preheat the oven to 375°F.

Heat a sauté pan to medium hot (see Note), add 2 tablespoons of the olive oil, then add the onion, fennel, carrots, zucchini, ¼ teaspoon salt, and 1 teaspoon herbes de Provence. Stir occasionally for at most 3 minutes, then set pan aside.

Place the trout in a large ovenproof dish, and rub with the remaining 2 tablespoons olive oil, ½ teaspoon salt, and 1 tablespoon herbes de Provence. Add the garlic to the inside of the trout.

Pour the partially cooked vegetables into the baking dish alongside the trout. Bake 25 to 30 minutes, or until the fish reaches 145–150°F.

To fillet the trout, place the fish on its side with the belly facing away from you. Start a small cut on the top side of the backbone just behind the head. Insert a filleting knife or other sharp, thin blade horizontally into this groove toward the belly of the fish and run the knife down the length of the fish, staying just above the backbone. Finish by slicing through the section at the base of the tail. You now have a clean, meaty fillet. Make a cut through the spine near the tail, then lift the spine and smaller bones out all in one piece. This will let you cut away the fillets from the other side of the fish. Next, place each fillet skin side down and pick out any bones along the belly of the fish that you find.

NOTE: The vegetables will take longer to bake than the trout. You can sauté the vegetables for 3 minutes to speed up their baking time, or skip this step and start baking the vegetables 15 minutes in advance, then adding the trout.

Sautéed Sole with Olive Oil, Parsley, and Green Onions

There is a mantra in Mediterranean Method cooking: If the ingredients are fresh, you don't have to do too much to them to make them delicious. The fishmonger at the market today sold me sole and urged me not to bathe it in too many other flavors—she wanted to be sure I'd really appreciate the deliciousness of this delicate fish. Once again, however, remember that freshness is the key.

This is delicious served with sautéed spinach, with extra garlic and olive oil and a dash of lemon—better to have the garlic on the side dish than on the sole, as it can overpower the delicate flavor.

PREP AND COOKING TIME: 20 minutes | SERVES 2

3 tablespoons extra-virgin olive oil

10 ounces sole fillets

¼ teaspoon sea salt

6 green onions, trimmed and left whole

1 teaspoon dried parsley (or 2 tablespoons finely chopped fresh)

1 organic lemon, half sliced and half juiced

Heat a sauté pan to medium hot and add the olive oil. Add the fish and salt, then lay in the green onions alongside the fish, cover, and sauté for about 4 minutes on the first side, turning once carefully. Sprinkle half the parsley on each side of sole. Tilt the pan occasionally to coat the fish and continue to cook until the second side flakes with a fork, another 3 to 4 minutes.

Carefully remove the fillets from the pan and place on a platter along with the green onions. Serve with lemon slices and drizzled with a little lemon juice.

Shrimp Kebabs

Grilling fish or meat with vegetables on a skewer is easy. When you marinate the animal protein in an acidic solution, you get the added benefit of avoiding most of the carcinogens that come with grilling at high heat. In this case, the acid is citrus, but you could also use vinegar or a balsamic vinaigrette.

PREP TIME: 15 minutes | MARINATING TIME: 15 minutes | GRILLING TIME: 15 minutes | SERVES 2

MARINADE

3 tablespoons avocado oil or almond oil

2 tablespoons fresh lemon juice

1 teaspoon paprika

1 teaspoon dried thyme

½ teaspoon sea salt

¼ teaspoon ground black pepper

⅛ teaspoon cayenne (optional)

4 medium garlic cloves, minced

SHRIMP AND VEGETABLES

12 ounces large shrimp, peeled and deveined

1 large red bell pepper, cored, seeded, and cut into 1-inch pieces

6 (2-inch) medium portobello or other button mushrooms, sliced in half

½ medium red onion, cut into quarters and separated into thin layers

12 fresh cherry tomatoes

SALAD

2 tablespoons extra-virgin olive oil

1 tablespoon red wine vinegar

½ teaspoon Dijon mustard

2 cups mixed greens

Preheat the grill to 450°F, or turn on the broiler to medium-high. Use 6 metal or wooden skewers; if using wooden skewers, soak them in water for 30 minutes before using.

Combine the marinade ingredients in a medium bowl with the shrimp, bell pepper, mushrooms, and red onion. Let marinate for 15 minutes, stirring occasionally.

Grease the skewers with oil, using a paper towel. On 4 skewers, alternate the red pepper, onion, mushrooms, and tomatoes. On 2 skewers, thread the shrimp, folding it in half so the skewer passes through each twice. (If you have leftover vegetables, you can grill them separately, without skewers.)

Grill or broil the vegetable skewers first, for 5 minutes, then add the shrimp skewers, turning all the skewers every 4 to 5 minutes for an additional 10 to 12 minutes, until the shrimp are pink and cooked. (See Note.)

Meanwhile, whisk together the olive oil, vinegar, and mustard, then toss with the greens and arrange on serving plates. Serve the kebabs atop the salads.

NOTE: A challenge with kebabs is using ingredients that cook for the same amount of time. The shrimp take 9 to 10 minutes on the grill, and the vegetables about 5 minutes longer. The easiest solution is to start grilling the vegetable skewers about 5 minutes sooner, then add the shrimp.

POULTRY DINNERS

Roasted Chicken with Mediterranean Herbs

Roast chicken doesn't have to be slathered in the standard American gravy to be good! Let herbs do the work of bringing out the delicious flavors. This dish is very quick and easy to prepare. Pop it in the oven and enjoy a delightfully flavored roasted chicken in 70 minutes.

PREP TIME: 15 minutes | ROASTING TIME: 1 hour, 10 minutes | SERVES 4

1 cage-free, organically fed small roasting chicken (about 3½ pounds)

½ teaspoon sea salt

½ teaspoon ground black pepper

1 tablespoon Italian herb seasoning

1 teaspoon minced fresh rosemary

2 tablespoons extra-virgin olive oil

Preheat the oven to 395°F.

Rinse the chicken, pat dry, and place in a roasting pan. Combine the salt, black pepper, herb seasoning, and rosemary in a small bowl. Massage the olive oil into the chicken, then sprinkle the herb mixture over and into the cavity.

Bake for 65 to 75 minutes, or until a meat thermometer stuck deep into the thigh reaches at least 165°F; the skin should be golden. Transfer the chicken to a cutting board and let it rest for 10 minutes before carving.

Moroccan Spiced Chicken

This dish offers fabulous Moroccan flavors and is packed with nutrients. I first tasted it at a rural farmhouse, seated on the floor, and we ate out of bowls with our fingers. I can still taste the delicious flavors.

PREP TIME: 20 minutes | COOKING TIME: 20 minutes | SERVES 4

2 tablespoons almond oil or avocado oil

8 skinless, boneless chicken thighs (1½ to 2 pounds total), sliced into 1-inch strips

⅔ teaspoon sea salt

1 (1-inch) piece fresh ginger, peeled and diced

1 medium onion, chopped

½ teaspoon ground coriander

¼ teaspoon ground cinnamon

1 red bell pepper, cored, seeded, and chopped

2 fresh medium tomatoes, chopped

1 (15-ounce) can garbanzo beans, rinsed and drained

4 medium garlic cloves, chopped

4 green onions, trimmed and chopped

½ cup pitted green olives

1 tablespoon toasted slivered almonds (or chopped pistachios)

1 teaspoon grated lemon rind

1 cup fresh herbs (cilantro, parsley, and/or mint)

Fresh mint sprigs

Heat a large skillet over medium-high heat, then add the oil, and then the chicken and salt. Stir occasionally for 6 to 8 minutes, or until the chicken is lightly browned. With a slotted spoon, transfer the chicken to a bowl.

Add the ginger and onion to the skillet, stir occasionally, and cook for 3 to 4 minutes, until translucent. Reduce the heat to medium, and add the coriander, cinnamon, bell pepper, and tomatoes. Scrape the bottom of the pan, then stir sporadically and cook for 3 minutes. Reduce the heat to a simmer, then add the beans, garlic, green onions, and olives. Stir the chicken back into the skillet, and cover to simmer another 4 to 5 minutes.

Meanwhile, heat a small sauté pan over medium heat, then add the almonds and toast for 3 to 4 minutes.

Stir the lemon rind and fresh herbs into the chicken, and simmer, covered, another 2 minutes. Transfer to serving plates and garnish with the toasted nuts and mint sprigs.

Duck with Port Wine Sauce and Mashed Sweet Potato

To my surprise, and in contrast to the United States, duck is featured on European restaurant menus and in European homes more often than chicken. Partly that is because of availability—in the U.S. it's more of a delicacy—but start spreading your wings (no pun intended) and pick up the duck when you see it. This recipe is easy to prepare and has a rich flavor. As when buying chicken, always look for organically raised, cage-free ducks.

PREP TIME: 20 minutes | COOKING TIME: 50 minutes | SERVES 2

2 medium sweet potatoes

2 (7- to 8-ounce) organic duck breasts

2 tablespoons avocado oil

$3/8$ teaspoon sea salt

$1/4$ teaspoon ground black pepper

2 teaspoons minced fresh thyme (or 1 teaspoon dried)

1 cup port wine

2 teaspoons extra-virgin olive oil

$1/2$ teaspoon ground cinnamon

$1/2$ cup unsweetened almond milk, warmed (or low-fat cow's milk)

Preheat the oven to 400°F. Pierce each sweet potato several times with the tines of a fork. Place the sweet potatoes on a rimmed baking sheet lined with foil. Bake until tender, 40 to 50 minutes.

Meanwhile, with a small sharp knife, score the duck skin in a crosshatch pattern. In a large bowl, combine the duck breasts, avocado oil, $1/4$ teaspoon salt, the black pepper, and thyme. Marinate for 5–10 minutes, stirring occasionally.

In a small saucepan over medium-low heat, combine the wine and $1/8$ teaspoon salt. Heat to a gentle boil, then reduce to low heat and simmer until reduced to $1/4$ cup, thickening to syrup, about 25 minutes. Keep warm.

Heat a medium sauté pan over medium-high. Place the duck skin side down in the pan and add the avocado oil and herbs. Cover and cook for 5 to 6 minutes, then turn and cook on the other side for another 4 to 5 minutes. Check the temperature; USDA recommendation for duck breast is an internal temperature of 170°F (medium to well done), although restaurants typically serve duck medium-rare, cooking it only to 140–145°F. Let rest for 3 to 5 minutes, then thinly slice. Keep warm.

Meanwhile, scoop the flesh out of the sweet potatoes and place in a food processor along with the olive oil, cinnamon, and almond milk. Purée until smooth. Spoon the purée onto plates, fan the duck slices over the sweet potato purée, then drizzle the port sauce over all and serve.

Chicken Breast with Pesto and Mixed Greens

This is a simple, flavorful recipe that might just become a go-to weeknight dinner. You can make this with chicken thighs, legs, or wings, but be sure to use cage-free, organic-fed chicken. Add other vegetables to the salad as you like.

PREP TIME: 15 minutes | SERVES 2

2 tablespoons avocado oil

10 ounces skinless, boneless chicken breast, sliced into 1-inch strips

¼ teaspoon salt

¼ teaspoon ground black pepper

2 tablespoons pesto sauce, store-bought or homemade (see page 227)

2 tablespoons extra-virgin olive oil

1 tablespoon red wine vinegar

4 cups mixed greens

2 cups quartered jarred artichoke hearts, packed in water or olive oil, drained

Heat a sauté pan over medium-high heat, then add the avocado oil, and then the chicken, salt, and black pepper. Cook, turning occasionally, until lightly browned, about 8 to 10 minutes. Set aside.

In a saucepan, simmer the pesto sauce.

In a large bowl, whisk together the olive oil and vinegar, then add the mixed greens and artichoke hearts. Toss well. Transfer the salad to individual plates and add the sautéed chicken strips, then drizzle the pesto sauce over all and serve.

Mediterranean Turkey Stew

Turkey—always available in the United States—is showing up commonly now in supermarkets and on restaurant menus throughout the Mediterranean region. Take your turkey up a notch with this recipe—it combines classic Mediterranean flavors in an easy-to-prepare format.

PREP TIME: 30–40 minutes | SERVES 4

2 tablespoons avocado oil

1 pound cage-free, organic ground turkey (from thigh and leg meat)

1 medium onion, chopped

½ teaspoon sea salt

¼ teaspoon ground black pepper

1 teaspoon Italian herb seasoning

2 tablespoons dry red wine

2 medium zucchini, quartered lengthwise and cut into ½-inch half-moons

2 tablespoons extra-virgin olive oil

1 medium red bell pepper, cored, seeded, and chopped

1 tablespoon balsamic vinegar

4 fresh medium tomatoes, chopped

3 garlic cloves, minced

1 (15-ounce) can garbanzo beans, rinsed and drained

¼ to ½ teaspoon hot sauce (optional)

Heat a large sauté pan over medium-high heat, then add the avocado oil, then the turkey, stirring occasionally, and sauté for 5 to 8 minutes until lightly browned. With a slotted spoon to keep the oil in the pan, remove the turkey and set aside.

In the same pan, immediately add the onion, salt, black pepper, and Italian herbs and sauté for 2 to 3 minutes, until the onion starts to soften. Add the wine and stir the bottom of the pan to deglaze. Reduce the heat to medium, then add the zucchini and olive oil, and cook 2 to 3 minutes, stirring occasionally. Add the bell pepper, balsamic vinegar, and tomatoes, then stir in the turkey and add the garlic and beans. Cover and simmer for 8 minutes. Taste, and add your favorite hot sauce, if desired. Serve immediately.

VEGETARIAN DINNERS

Roasted Garbanzo Beans, Bell Peppers, and Cauliflower with a Lemon-Yogurt Sauce

Here is a quick and easy dish, loaded with healthy ingredients. Curry spices reduce inflammation and have essential health benefits. If you'd like a bit of heat in the dish, add your favorite chili sauce or a dash of cayenne.

PREP TIME: 15 minutes | COOKING TIME: 35–40 minutes | SERVES 4

¼ cup extra-virgin olive oil

2 teaspoons curry spice

1 teaspoon paprika

¼ teaspoon cayenne (optional)

½ teaspoon sea salt

¼ teaspoon ground black pepper

1 large cauliflower, trimmed and cut into bite-sized pieces

1 medium onion, sliced into thin strips

1 medium green bell pepper, cored, seeded, and cut into 1-inch pieces

1 medium red bell pepper, cored, seeded, and cut into 1-inch pieces

2 (15-ounce) cans garbanzo beans, rinsed and drained

1 cup organic plain low-fat yogurt

2 tablespoons lemon juice

1 teaspoon dillweed (or 1 tablespoon minced fresh)

¼ cup fresh mint, finely chopped

Preheat the oven to 375°F.

In a large bowl, whisk together the olive oil, curry spices, paprika, cayenne if using, salt, and black pepper. Toss in the cauliflower, onion, bell peppers, and beans. Spread the mixture on a lipped baking sheet, and bake for 35 to 40 minutes, or until vegetables are tender.

Meanwhile, combine the yogurt, lemon juice, dill, and mint in a bowl.

Spoon the roasted vegetables onto serving plates, and drizzle the yogurt sauce over. Serve at once.

Ratatouille with Cannellini Beans

My family loves this fragrant and delicious recipe from the South of France, and lucky for all of us, it's packed with nutrients. Ratatouille can be served hot or cold, and usually tastes better when served the next day. With the beans included, it makes a whole meal, or you can skip the beans and serve this as a side dish.

PREP TIME: 10 minutes | COOKING TIME: 20 minutes | SERVES 4 as main dish

1 medium Italian eggplant, ends trimmed, cut into 1-inch cubes

¼ cup extra-virgin olive oil

1 medium sweet onion, finely chopped

½ teaspoon sea salt

¼ teaspoon ground black pepper

1 teaspoon fines herbes (or Italian herb seasoning)

3 small zucchini, cut into ½-inch cubes (about 2½ cups)

2 small yellow squash, cut into ½-inch cubes (about 2 cups)

2 tablespoons dry red wine

3 fresh medium tomatoes, chopped (about 2½ cups)

4 medium garlic cloves, minced

1 tablespoon finely chopped Italian flat-leaf parsley

1 teaspoon minced fresh rosemary

1 tablespoon finely chopped fresh basil

1 (15-ounce) can cannellini beans, rinsed and drained

⅛ teaspoon paprika or cayenne

Fresh parsley, basil, and/or thyme, for garnish

Heat a large sauté pan over medium-high heat, then add the eggplant and about 2 tablespoons of water; cook for 2 to 3 minutes, stirring occasionally. When the water has evaporated, reduce the heat to medium and add 2 tablespoons of the olive oil; sauté another 2 to 3 minutes, until the eggplant is tender.

Meanwhile, heat a large saucepan over medium heat and add the remaining 2 tablespoons olive oil, then add the onion, salt, black pepper, and fines herbes. Sauté for 2 to 3 minutes, or until the onion is soft and translucent. Add the zucchini, yellow squash, eggplant, and the wine, and stir. Cover and cook for 3 to 4 minutes, until the vegetables soften, stirring occasionally. Reduce the heat to low, and add the tomatoes, garlic, and fresh herbs. Cover, add the beans, and simmer for 10 minutes, or until squash softens and the flavors blend. Taste and add either paprika or cayenne as desired.

Garnish with the fresh herbs and serve.

Spanish Tortilla (Omelet)

This sounds fancy, but it's really a humble (and delicious) omelet! Enjoy it for lunch, dinner, or as part of a spread with other small plates (as the Spanish do with tapas). Though I generally avoid potatoes—due to their high glycemic (sugar) load, in this dish they do provide a good source of fiber and nutrients.

A way to lower the glycemic load is to select small fingerling 1- to 2-inch potatoes, or use a smaller portion of potatoes, or boil and refrigerate the cooked potatoes in advance. It takes a bit of planning, and involves a couple extra steps, but if you have the patience, it's worth it.

PREP AND COOKING TIME: 30 minutes | SERVES 2

4 tablespoons extra-virgin olive oil

1¼ cups (⅓ pound) baby potatoes, cut into ¼-inch slices (see Tip)

1 small sweet onion, thinly sliced

½ medium red bell pepper, cored, seeded, and diced

5 cage-free, organic large eggs

¼ teaspoon sea salt

¼ teaspoon ground black pepper

¼ cup fresh Italian flat-leaf parsley, finely chopped

COOK'S TIP: Baby potatoes with the skin that are boiled and chilled have a much lower glycemic load than regular peeled potatoes that are baked or sautéed, and they still taste great. Simply boil the sliced potatoes in advance until al dente (7–9 minutes), drain, then refrigerate for 4 to 24 hours, until well chilled. When ready to serve, heat along with the oil and onion as noted here, but you'll only need to sauté them for 5 minutes, as they are already cooked.

Heat a medium sauté pan or skillet over medium-low heat. Add 2 tablespoons of the olive oil, then add the potatoes, onion, and bell pepper, then cover and simmer for about 15 minutes, stirring the potatoes and onion every 5 minutes or so until potatoes are soft and tender.

Meanwhile, whisk the eggs with the salt, pepper, and parsley in a large bowl.

Spoon the potato mixture into the bowl with the eggs and mix well. With a paper towel, wipe the bottom of the sauté pan to remove any sticky material.

Heat the same sauté pan over medium heat, then add the remaining 2 tablespoons olive oil. Pour the egg and potato mixture into the pan, cover, reduce the heat to medium-low, and cook for 4 to 5 minutes. When eggs are nearly set and the underside is lightly golden, invert the omelet onto a plate, then slide it back into the pan and cook a few more minutes. When the underside is golden, slide it back onto a plate and serve.

Falafel Lettuce Wraps

Falafel appears to have come from Egypt and originally was made with fava beans. In recent times, and with falafel's growing popularity, it is now made in the United States mostly with garbanzo beans. Either way, falafel is a great source of nutrients and protein, and is very heart healthy. Falafel is traditionally served with pita bread (basically a big load of white flour). Using cabbage or lettuce wraps is a much healthier alternative; although it's a little bit messier, it's still fun to eat and the wrap adds a nice crunch. There are dozens of condiments that can go with falafel. Here I have picked four basics to keep it simple: hummus, tzatziki (yogurt-cucumber sauce), tahini, and salsa.

BEAN SOAKING TIME: 8–12 hours | PREP TIME: 60 minutes | SERVES 4–6 (makes 24 small or 12 large)

¾ pound (about 2 cups) dried garbanzo beans

2 tablespoons salt

1 medium onion, finely chopped

¾ cup fresh Italian flat-leaf parsley

4 medium garlic cloves, peeled

¾ cup fresh cilantro

1 teaspoon ground cumin

½ teaspoon ground coriander

¼ teaspoon ground black pepper

¼ teaspoon cayenne

⅛ teaspoon ground cinnamon

2 to 4 tablespoons chickpea flour

8 to 12 large green cabbage leaves (or large Bibb or Boston lettuce leaves)

1½ cups avocado oil or grapeseed oil (see Note)

½ cup tzatziki (page 228)

½ cup jarred salsa (tomato-based, with no or minimal sugar added)

½ cup hummus (page 229)

¼ to ⅓ cup tahini

Place the beans into a large bowl and cover them with about 3 inches of water; add the salt. Let soak overnight at room temperature; they will double in size, making about 4 cups. Drain and rinse well.

Pour the soaked beans into a food processor or blender, working in batches if necessary. Add the onion, parsley, garlic, cilantro, cumin, coriander, black pepper, cayenne, cinnamon, and flour. Process until mostly smooth, scraping down the sides as needed; it should still be a bit chunky—you don't want it totally smooth, like hummus.

Preheat the oven to 250°F

Using wet hands, form 2 tablespoons each of the falafel mixture into balls. If they fall apart, add a bit more flour to make them stick together. (You also may need to process the mixture a bit finer.) Then flatten the balls so they are patties about 2 inches across and 1 inch thick. (There is a falafel scoop that does this for you if you have one.)

If using cabbage leaves, lightly steam the leaves in a large steamer for 3 to 4 minutes.

Heat the avocado oil in a deep 6-inch-wide saucepan to 370°F over medium-high heat; do not let the oil burn or smoke. Use a thermometer to monitor the oil temperature while frying and be prepared to reduce the temperature as needed (best is in a range of 360–375°F).

Test a falafel by dropping it into the hot oil and seeing that it holds together and fries well. If so, continue to fry the falafel for 2 to 3 minutes per side, until golden brown. (If you don't have a deep-frying thermometer and the falafel cooks quicker than this, reduce the temperature; if the outside cooks too quickly, the inside will be raw. Similarly, if they are not cooking quickly enough, you'll need to increase the temperature a bit.) Use a slotted spoon to remove the falafel and continue to deep-fry. You can keep the cooked falafel warm on a tray in a warmed oven.

Have serving bowls ready with the tzaziki, salsa, hummus, and tahini. Have lots of paper napkins ready.

Pile the falafel on a platter. For each falafel wrap, add 1 to 2 tablespoons hummus, 2 to 3 falafel, 1 to 2 tablespoons tzatziki, and 1 to 2 tablespoons salsa, and then drizzle 1 teaspoon of tahini over all and wrap up the cabbage leaf.

NOTE: Each falafel patty absorbs about ½ teaspoon of oil, so with 24 patties, that is a total of 3–4 tablespoons of oil, which is why selecting a healthy oil is so important here. Also note: Don't try making this with canned beans—here is a case when you need to soak dried beans.

Black-Eyed Pea and Pomegranate Salad

Black-eyed peas have come to us from Africa and are a popular food in Egypt and along North Africa. There, they are commonly served with mixed herbs, walnuts, and pomegranate seeds, as in this quick-to-prepare and delicious salad. You don't want mushy black-eyed peas, which you get sometimes with the canned versions, so it's best to make this from either dried or fresh peas and cook them until al dente. Traditionally, this recipe is prepared with pomegranate molasses, adding a liquid sugar—it's better as I've done here, adding an extra portion of delicious pomegranate seeds!

PREP TIME: 15–20 minutes | SERVES 4

4 cups cooked black-eyed peas, rinsed and drained (see Note)

1 cup arugula (rocket), trimmed and chopped

½ cup Italian flat-leaf parsley, finely chopped

¼ cup fresh mint, finely chopped

2 celery stalks, finely chopped

3 green onions, trimmed and finely chopped

½ cup walnuts, finely chopped

¾ to 1 cup pomegranate seeds

6 tablespoons extra-virgin olive oil

3 to 4 tablespoons fresh lemon juice

½ teaspoon sea salt

¼ teaspoon ground black pepper

Combine the peas, arugula, parsley, mint, celery, green onions, walnuts, and pomegranate seeds in a serving bowl.

Whisk together the olive oil, lemon juice to taste, the salt, and black pepper. Pour over the peas and toss to coat well, then serve.

NOTE: To cook dried black-eyed peas, pour the peas into a saucepan, cover with water, and bring to a boil for 2 to 3 minutes. Remove the pot from the heat and allow to stand for 60 to 90 minutes. Drain and replace with fresh water, then bring to a boil a second time and simmer for about 60 minutes, until tender.

To prepare fresh black-eyed peas, add them to a saucepan, cover with water, bring to a gentle boil, then simmer for 60 to 70 minutes, until tender but still al dente.

SIDE DISHES

Grilled Asparagus with Olive Oil and Lemon

This is simple to prepare and loaded with healthy nutrients. With the Mediterranean Method, you can grill nearly any vegetable and toss it with olive oil, lemon juice, and garlic for a terrific side dish. When buying asparagus, look for thick stalks, which are more tender.

PREP TIME: 10–15 minutes | SERVES 2

16 spears (about 1 pound) asparagus, trimmed

2 tablespoons extra-virgin olive oil

2 medium garlic cloves, minced

1 tablespoon fresh lemon juice

¼ teaspoon sea salt

Preheat the grill to 400°F.

Grill the asparagus, turning occasionally, until lightly browned, 5 to 8 minutes.

Meanwhile, heat a small pan over medium heat, then add the olive oil and garlic and sauté for 1 to 2 minutes, or until garlic is cooked (don't let the garlic brown). Add lemon juice and set aside.

Toss the grilled asparagus with the flavored oil and salt, and serve.

Roasted Beet, Leek, and Kale Salad

Dark green and deep red—beautiful colors on the plate, and full of polyphenols, not to mention delicious. And a bonus benefit: These vegetables can easily be roasted a day in advance. Simply toss with dressing before serving.

PREP TIME: 20 minutes | ROASTING TIME: 35–45 minutes | SERVES 4

4 medium beets, peeled and sliced

2 medium leeks, trimmed, washed carefully, and white base and first inch of green chopped

4 tablespoons extra-virgin olive oil

½ teaspoon sea salt

¼ teaspoon ground black pepper

1 teaspoon Italian herb seasoning

12 medium kale leaves, ribs cut out, leafy part sliced into large bite-sized pieces

¼ cup pistachios, chopped

2 tablespoons crumbled feta cheese (optional)

DRESSING

4 tablespoons extra-virgin olive oil

2 tablespoons fresh lemon juice

1 tablespoon honey

1 medium garlic clove, diced

1 teaspoon dried oregano

⅛ teaspoon sea salt

Preheat the oven to 395°F.

Toss the beets and leeks in a medium bowl with 2 tablespoons of the olive oil, ¼ teaspoon of the salt, the black pepper, and Italian seasoning. Stir to coat well. Arrange the beets and leeks on a rimmed baking sheet and roast for 35 to 45 minutes, until tender but still firm.

Meanwhile, toss the kale in a small bowl with the remaining 2 tablespoons olive oil and ¼ teaspoon salt. Spread on a baking sheet. Roast for 10 to 15 minutes, until crisp.

Heat a small sauté pan over medium heat, then add the pistachios, stirring frequently until warmed through; don't allow the nuts to brown.

Whisk together the dressing ingredients in a bowl.

When ready to serve, place the kale on a serving platter, drizzle the dressing over and toss gently, then add the beets and leeks and garnish with the nuts and cheese, if using. Serve warm or at room temperature.

Za'atar Sautéed Fennel and Spinach with Farro

Za'atar is a special spice blend from the eastern Mediterranean region and the Middle East. It consists of roasted sesame seeds, thyme, sumac, oregano, and marjoram, and it can be served with a variety of dishes—including the main protein you serve with this side dish. Farro is a whole-grain form of an ancient type of wheat, so if you are gluten sensitive, substitute quinoa and/or wild rice. To transform this into a full vegetarian meal, add 2 cups of cooked beans.

PREP TIME: 25–30 minutes | SERVES 4

1 cup semi-pearled farro

2 tablespoons extra-virgin olive oil

1 medium red onion, sliced in half and then finely sliced

1 medium fennel bulb, trimmed, halved lengthwise, and sliced thinly crosswise

1 tablespoon Za'atar spice blend (or ¾ teaspoon each of dried thyme, dried oregano, dried marjoram, and crushed sesame seeds)

¼ teaspoon sea salt

4 cups fresh spinach

1 teaspoon grated lemon zest

1 tablespoon fresh lemon juice

Bring a pot of salted water to a boil. Add the farro and simmer for 15 to 20 minutes, until tender. Drain and set aside.

Heat a large sauté pan over medium heat, then add the olive oil and onion, stir, and heat for 1 minute. Add the fennel, Za'atar, and salt and heat for 5 minutes, stirring occasionally, until fennel is tender. Add the spinach and heat with a sporadic stir until it wilts, then add the lemon zest, lemon juice, and farro. Cook with an occasional stir for 2 to 3 minutes and serve.

Sautéed Kale with Garlic and Lemon Zest

Mediterranean vegetable side dishes are often simple to make and delicious, using extra-virgin olive oil at medium-low heat, plus garlic and lemon—a wonderful combination. You can substitute spinach, broccoli, green beans, and other green vegetables for the kale—the key is to use fresh produce.

PREP TIME: 10–15 minutes | SERVES 2

3 tablespoons extra-virgin olive oil

½ medium onion, thinly sliced

5 cups chopped fresh kale

¼ teaspoon sea salt

½ teaspoon dried thyme or fines herbes

2 medium garlic cloves, minced

1 teaspoon grated lemon zest

2 teaspoons fresh lemon juice

Heat a large sauté pan over medium heat, then add the olive oil, then the onion and cook for 2 minutes, or until the onion softens.

Add the kale, salt, and thyme, stirring occasionally for 2 to 3 minutes, until the kale starts to wilt. Reduce the heat to a simmer, add the garlic and lemon zest, and cook another 1 to 2 minutes with a sporadic stir. Add lemon juice and then serve.

Gigantes and Chard
with Roasted Tomato, Onion, and Garlic

Gigantes are also called fava beans (but large ones). If you can't find large fava beans, select extra-large lima or broad beans. The bean cooking time will depend on the type of bean you select and how long you soak them. Or use 2 (15-ounce) cans of beans to cut the prep time here down to 50 minutes; just simmer the canned beans in 1 cup water for 5 minutes while the tomatoes are roasting, then drain and continue with the recipe.

BEAN PREPARATION: Soaking, 10–12 hours; simmering 1-2 hours | PREP TIME: 20 minutes
COOKING TIME: 40 minutes | SERVES 4

1 cup large dried fava beans

2 cups low-sodium vegetable broth

4 cups water

5 tablespoons extra-virgin olive oil

4 fresh medium tomatoes, chopped

4 medium garlic cloves, chopped

1 medium sweet onion, chopped

¼ teaspoon sea salt

¼ teaspoon ground black pepper

1 teaspoon dried oregano

4 cups chopped chard (including red stems, if desired)

Place the dried beans in a large bowl and add enough water to cover by 2 inches. Soak overnight (preferably 10–12 hours). Drain.

Place the soaked beans in a large pot with the broth and water. Bring to a gentle boil, then simmer over low heat for 1½ to 2½ hours, until the beans have softened, but are still slightly al dente.

Preheat the oven to 375°F.

Using a baking sheet with rimmed edges, combine 4 tablespoons of the olive oil, the tomatoes, garlic, onion, salt, black pepper, and oregano; toss to coat the tomatoes well. Roast for 40 minutes, or until the tomato liquid has mostly evaporated and onion and tomato pieces are baked.

Just before serving, heat a large skillet over medium heat, then add the remaining tablespoon of olive oil and the chard; sauté for 2 to 3 minutes, until wilted.

In a large serving bowl, combine the beans, roasted tomatoes, and chard. Stir to combine, and serve.

Stuffed Roasted Eggplant

I've enjoyed stuffed eggplant throughout the Mediterranean region, in a half dozen countries and prepared in many different ways. My favorite involves roasting the eggplant and then stuffing it, thereby improving its flavor and texture. This version can be served by itself as a light meal or as a side dish with fish or poultry.

PREP TIME: 20 minutes | BAKING TIME: 60 minutes | SERVES 4

2 medium to large eggplants (about 3 pounds total), trimmed and sliced in half lengthwise

4 tablespoons extra-virgin olive oil

½ medium onion, finely chopped

½ teaspoon sea salt

¼ teaspoon ground black pepper

1 teaspoon dried oregano

2 tablespoons dry white wine

2 fresh medium tomatoes, chopped

¼ teaspoon red pepper flakes

4 medium garlic cloves, minced

1 cup (⅔ of 15-ounce can) cannellini beans, rinsed and drained

½ cup Italian flat-leaf parsley, finely chopped

2 tablespoons slivered almonds

¼ cup grated Parmesan cheese (optional)

Preheat the oven to 375°F.

With a sharp paring knife, score the eggplant halves 1 inch deep in a diamond pattern. Brush the cuts with 1 tablespoon of the olive oil. Place cut side down in a greased ovenproof dish and roast for 40 minutes.

Meanwhile, heat a sauté pan over medium heat, then add the remaining 3 tablespoons olive oil, then the onion, salt, black pepper, and oregano and sauté for 3 minutes, stirring occasionally. Add the wine and stir to loosen particles on pan bottom, then add the tomatoes, red pepper flakes, and garlic. Lower the heat and simmer for 3 minutes. Mix in the beans and parsley and set aside.

With a spoon and/or paring knife, scoop out the eggplant flesh, creating a hollow for stuffing. Discard any heavily seeded eggplant parts. Mince the remaining eggplant pulp and add to the skillet mixture. Stir to combine.

Stuff the eggplant halves with the vegetable and bean mixture, packing it firmly into each and making a small mound. Sprinkle on top with the almonds and then the grated cheese, if using. Return the eggplants to the baking dish and bake another 20 minutes to heat through. Serve.

DESSERTS

Blueberry Ricotta Cheesecake

The Italians know dessert. Substitute any berry for the topping in this recipe, but I like organic blueberries. Those, together with the orange rind in the filling, is a combination that provides valuable nutrients and a unique flavor. The almonds add healthy fats, and the sour cream gives a probiotic boost.

PREP TIME: 20 minutes | BAKING TIME: 60 minutes | SERVES 12

CRUST

⅔ cup almond flour

1 cup almonds, finely chopped

1 teaspoon ground cinnamon

1 tablespoon honey

½ cup ghee (clarified butter), plus more for greasing the pie plate

FILLING

16 ounces part-skim ricotta

1 cup honey (or xylitol)

1 teaspoon vanilla extract

2 tablespoons almond flour

2 teaspoons grated orange zest

¼ teaspoon sea salt

6 cage-free, organic large eggs, lightly beaten

TOPPING

½ cup organic low-fat sour cream

1 cup blueberries

Preheat the oven to 350°F.

In a medium bowl, combine the almond flour, chopped almonds, and cinnamon. Mix in the honey and ghee. Grease a 9-inch pie plate (or 8- to 9-inch springform pan) and press and spread the crust mixture into and up the sides.

In a mixer, beat the ricotta, honey, vanilla, almond flour, 1 teaspoon of the orange zest, and the salt until smooth. Add the eggs and beat on low until smooth. Pour the filling into the crust.

Place the pie plate on a baking sheet and bake the crust and filling until the center is set, about 60 minutes. Remove and let stand on a wire rack for 10 minutes.

Spoon the sour cream over the top, then sprinkle on the blueberries and garnish with the remaining teaspoon of orange rind. Refrigerate at least 2 hours, or overnight.

Pears Poached with Wine and Cinnamon

The French know dessert, too! In this delicious preparation, the tartness of the yogurt, the sweetness and delicate flavors of the pear, and the bitterness of the dark chocolate are an unbeatable combination. You can substitute many other fruits, such as apples, peaches, or apricots. For a special occasion, you could substitute organic vanilla ice cream for the yogurt. And if you are dairy-free, use a dairy-free form of yogurt, such as one made from coconut milk.

PREP TIME: 15 minutes | COOKING TIME: 30 minutes | CHILLING TIME: 1–24 hours | SERVES 4

1½ cups dry white wine (Chardonnay, Chablis, or Sauvignon Blanc)

1 cinnamon stick

1 teaspoon vanilla extract

1 tablespoon fresh lemon juice

⅛ teaspoon sea salt

¼ teaspoon ground cardamom

4 tablespoons honey (or xylitol)

4 ripe Bosc pears, cored and quartered lengthwise

4 tablespoons organic plain low-fat Greek yogurt

4 (1-ounce) pieces dark chocolate (at least 74% cacao)

In a medium pot, combine the wine, cinnamon stick, vanilla, lemon juice, salt, cardamom, and honey. Bring to a gentle boil, then simmer for 5 minutes. Add the pears, return to a gentle boil, then simmer, turning pears occasionally, until pears are tender, about 15 minutes. Remove the pears with a slotted spoon and set aside.

Bring the remaining liquid to a gentle boil, and continue to cook on medium heat for 15 minutes, allowing the sauce to thicken; be careful not to overheat and burn the sauce. Discard the cinnamon stick.

In a serving dish, distribute the pears into the bowl, then drizzle the sauce over the pears. (Optionally, you can pour the sauce through a fine-mesh screen to remove any particulate matter.) Refrigerate the bowls at least 1 hour and up to 24 hours.

Just before serving, add 1 tablespoon of yogurt to each bowl, place a piece of dark chocolate on the side, and serve.

Grilled Figs with Port

Summertime in the Mediterranean region means figs are in season. Luscious and ubiquitous, they are an amazing treat. If you see fresh figs in your grocery store, try this recipe!

PREP TIME: 15 minutes | SERVES 2

Cooking spray

1 pound fresh purple figs, sliced in half

2 tablespoons port wine

2 tablespoons half-and-half (or dairy-free half-and-half)

⅛ teaspoon vanilla extract

Preheat a grill or a broiler. Lightly cover the grill with a sheet of aluminum foil and lightly coat with cooking spray, or line a broiler pan with the foil.

Grill or broil the figs for 2 to 3 minutes per side, until lightly browned.

Meanwhile, whisk together the wine, half-and-half, and vanilla.

Place the grilled figs in small serving bowls, pour the wine sauce on top, and serve.

Peaches and Berries
with Muscatel Wine and Mint

Here is a lovely dessert, very easy and quick to prepare, and my guests love it. If you have trouble finding Muscatel (Moscatel), substitute a Sauterne or other sweet wine (or port). You can also serve dessert with a small glass (2-ounce serving) of Muscatel. Feel free to use a variety of other fruits—whatever is in season, such as apples, pineapple, mango, or cantaloupe.

PREP TIME: 10 minutes | CHILLING TIME: 20 minutes | SERVES 2

2 medium peaches, pitted and cut into
bite-sized pieces

1 cup mixed berries (raspberries,
blueberries, strawberries, blackberries)

2 tablespoons Muscatel sweet wine
(or port or other sweet wine)

2 tablespoons minced fresh mint

In a serving bowl, combine the peaches, berries, wine, and mint. Refrigerate at least 20 minutes before serving.

Berry and Apple Crumble

This dessert is simple to make, popular with guests, and loaded with brain- and heart-friendly nutrients. You can use frozen berries or enjoy them fresh if in season, although fresh strawberries are better in a crumble like this than frozen. You can substitute any nuts you have in your pantry, and use whatever fruit is in season, such as peaches, cherries, or pears in place of the apple.

PREP TIME: 15 minutes | BAKING TIME: 15 minutes | SERVES 4

½ cup old-fashioned rolled oats

1 tablespoon ghee (clarified butter)

⅓ cup slivered almonds

⅓ cup chopped hazelnuts

⅓ cup unsweetened dried coconut

¼ cup port wine

2 tablespoons honey

1 teaspoon lemon zest

1 tablespoon fresh lemon juice

¼ teaspoon ground cinnamon

⅛ teaspoon sea salt

1/16 teaspoon cayenne

1 medium apple (such as Ambrosia, Pink Lady, Fuji)

2 cups fresh strawberries, hulled and quartered

1 cup fresh blueberries

1 cup fresh raspberries

Additional berries for serving

Whipped cream (optional)

Preheat the oven to 350°F.

Heat a medium skillet over medium-low heat, then add the oats and butter, and toast with a sporadic stir until the oats are lightly browned, 3 to 4 minutes. Add the almonds, hazelnuts, and coconut, and toast over low heat with an occasional stir for another 3 to 4 minutes.

Combine the port, honey, lemon zest and juice, cinnamon, salt, cayenne, and apple in a medium saucepan. Bring to a simmer and cook for 2 to 3 minutes. Stir in the berries, and remove from the heat.

Pour the berry sauce into a pie plate. Sprinkle the toasted oats and nuts on top. Bake for 15 minutes, or until bubbling. Allow to cool for 10 minutes, then serve warm, garnished with several fresh berries and, optionally, add a dollop of whipped cream.

SAUCES & DIPS

Pesto

Pesto is used widely as a condiment throughout the Mediterranean region, especially in Italy. This recipe is a rather classic preparation, but you can also include olives, roasted red bell peppers, and a variety of nuts.

PREP TIME: 15 minutes | MAKES 1 cup

4 medium garlic cloves, peel left on

¼ cup pine nuts

¼ cup almonds, preferably skinned

3 packed cups fresh basil leaves, stems and any brown leaves removed

½ teaspoon ground black pepper

½ cup extra-virgin olive oil

½ cup grated Parmesan cheese (1¾ ounces)

⅛ teaspoon fine sea salt

Heat a sauté pan over medium heat, and toast the garlic for 3 to 4 minutes, until warmed and very lightly browned. Remove from the heat and set aside to cool, then remove the skin and dice the garlic.

In a food processor, pulse the pine nuts and almonds for 15 seconds. Add the basil, toasted garlic, and black pepper and pulse another 15 seconds. With the food processor running, slowly pour in the olive oil until thoroughly mixed. Add the cheese and pulse until the pesto is smooth, 30 to 45 seconds. Add the salt, and pulse one last time.

Tzatziki

This is a delicious Greek yogurt sauce, used as a dip for raw vegetables or drizzled over vegetables or grilled chicken. Greek yogurt is essential—don't try this with regular yogurt or it will be too watery. The tzatziki will store in the refrigerator for several days. If you're dairy-free, this is a recipe you'll have to forgo; there really is no good substitute for the dairy here.

PREP TIME: 15–20 minutes | MAKES 3 cups

2 cups (16 ounces) organic plain low-fat Greek yogurt

1 small English cucumber, peeled, sliced in half lengthwise, seeded, and grated (see Note)

2 medium garlic cloves, minced

2 tablespoons fresh lemon juice

2 tablespoons extra-virgin olive oil

2 teaspoons grated lemon zest

3 tablespoons finely chopped fresh dill

½ teaspoon sea salt

¼ teaspoon ground black pepper

In a bowl, combine all the ingredients and stir until smooth. Cover and refrigerate for at least 30 minutes, then serve.

NOTE: It's easiest to grate the cucumber with a food processor, but it's simple enough to do with a hand grater, then allow it to drain in a sieve, pressing out excess liquid, before mixing with the yogurt.

Method Hummus

Many Americans are used to dipping pita bread into hummus, but a better Mediterranean style is to use vegetables instead. I like to garnish a bowl of hummus with diced tomato, black olives, and some crumbled feta, as it adds color and complementary flavors, and then dip with sliced cucumber, jicama, or other sliced vegetables.

PREP TIME: 30 minutes | MAKES about 1 cup

1 (15-ounce) can garbanzo beans (or 1¾ cups cooked; see Note), rinsed and drained

½ teaspoon baking soda

2 small garlic cloves, minced

¼ to ⅓ cup fresh lemon juice

¼ teaspoon ground cumin

½ teaspoon sea salt

¼ teaspoon ground black pepper

⅓ cup sesame tahini

¼ cup extra-virgin olive oil

2 to 4 tablespoons water

3 fresh cherry tomatoes, sliced in half

6 unpitted black olives

1 to 2 ounces feta cheese, cut into ½-inch cubes (about ½ cup)

NOTE: Hummus is best prepared with thoroughly cooked garbanzo beans. Canned beans are fine, but be sure to buy BPA-free ones. The critical step for a smooth hummus is to simmer the beans with baking soda to soften the skins. If you're using dried beans, soak them overnight and cook until tender; then simmer with baking soda as noted here.

In a large saucepan, combine the beans, baking soda, and enough water to cover the beans. Bring to a gentle boil, then simmer for 20 minutes. Pour through a strainer, rinse well, and set aside.

Place the garlic, lemon juice, cumin, salt, and black pepper in a food processor, and blend until smooth. Let sit for 10 minutes to allow the lemon flavor to blend with the garlic.

Add the tahini and 3 tablespoons of the olive oil to the food processor and blend until smooth, scraping the sides of the processor as needed. Then add the beans and process until well blended, scraping the sides of the processor again as needed. Add some water, 1 tablespoon at a time, until smooth.

When ready to serve, spread the hummus on a plate or place in a flat bowl, then stir in the remaining tablespoon of olive oil. Garnish with the cherry tomatoes, black olives, and feta.

References

1: A Whole-Foods Diet for the Whole Planet

Buettner, Dan. The island where people forget to die. *New York Times Magazine*, October 28, 2012.

Katz, D.L; Meller, S. Can we say what diet is best? *Annual Review of Public Health*, 2014; 35:83–103.

2: How to Eat: A New Mediterranean Diet

Berger, K.; Ajani, U.A.; et al. Light to moderate alcohol consumption and the risk of stroke among US male physicians. *New England Journal of Medicine*, 1999; 341:1557–64.

Faridi, Z.; et al. Acute dark chocolate and cocoa ingestion and endothelial function. *American Journal of Clinical Nutrition*, 2008; 88:58–63.

Foster, G.D.; Shantz, K.L.; et al. A randomized trial of the effects of an almond-enriched, hypocaloric diet in the treatment of obesity. *American Journal of Clinical Nutrition*, 2012, Aug.; 96(2):249–54.

Fraga, C.G. Cocoa, diabetes, and hypertension: should we eat more chocolate? *American Journal of Clinical Nutrition*, 2005; 81:541–42.

Grassi, D.; Lippi, C.; et al. Short-term administration of dark chocolate in followed by a significant increase in insulin sensitivity and a decrease in blood pressure in healthy persons. *American Journal of Clinical Nutrition*, 2005; 81:611–14.

Ibarrola-Jurado, N.; Bullo, M.; et al. Cross-sectional assessment of nut consumption and obesity, metabolic syndrome and other cardiometabolic risk factors: the PREDIMED study. *PLOS ONE*, 2013; 8(2):e57367.

Jenkins, D.J.A.; Kendall, C.W.C.; et al. Effect of legumes as part of a low glycemic index diet on glycemic control and cardiovascular risk factors in type 2 diabetes mellitus. *Archives of Internal Medicine*, 2012; 172:1653–60.

Martínez-González, M.A.; et al. Empirically-derived food patterns and the risk of total mortality and cardiovascular events in the PREDIMED study. *Clinical Nutrition*, 2015; 34(5):859–67.

Rein, D.; Paglieroni, T.G.; et al. Cocoa inhibits platelet activation and function. *American Journal of Clinical Nutrition*, 2000; 72:30–35.

Rimm, E.B.; Ellison, R.C. Alcohol in the Mediterranean diet. *American Journal of Clinical Nutrition*, 1995; 61:1378–82.

Rousseau, Bryant. Rosemary and time: an Italian recipe for longevity. *New York Times*, October 20, 2016.

Sabate, J.; et al. Effects of walnuts on serum lipoid levels and blood pressure in men. *New England Journal of Medicine*, 1993; 328:603–607.

Silagy, C.A.; Neil, H.A. A meta-analysis of the effect of garlic on blood pressure. *Journal of Hypertension*, 1994; 12:463–68.

Solomon, C.G.; Hu, F.B.; et al. Moderate alcohol consumption and risk of coronary heart disease among women with type 2 diabetes. *Circulation*, 2000; 102:494–99.

Spiller, G.A.; et al. Effects of plant-based diets high in raw or roasted almonds or almond butter on serum lipoproteins in humans. *Journal of the American College of Nutrition*, 2003; 22:195–200.

Steiner, M.; Khan, A.H.; et al. A double-blind crossover study in moderately hypercholesterol-emic men that compared the effect of aged garlic extract and placebo on blood lipids. *American Journal of Clinical Nutrition*, 1996; 64:866–70.

Taubert, D.; Roesen, R.; et al. Effects of low habitual cocoa intake on blood pressure and bioactive nitric oxide. *JAMA*, 2007; 298:49–60.

Thun, M.J.; Peto, R.; et al. Alcohol consumption and mortality among middle aged and elderly US adults. *New England Journal of Medicine*, 1997; 337; 1705–14.

Trichopoulou. A.; Bamia, C.; et al. Anatomy of health effects of Mediterranean diet: Greek EPIC prospective cohort study. *BMJ*, 2009; 338:b2337. doi:10.1136/bmj.b2337.

Turati, F.; et al. Glycemic load and coronary heart disease in a Mediterranean population: The EPIC Greek cohort study. *Nutrition, Metabolism & Cardiovascular Diseases*, 2015; 25:336e342.

Wan, Y.; et al. Effects of cocoa powder and dark chocolate on LDL oxidative susceptibility and prostaglandin concentrations in humans. *American Journal of Clinical Nutrition*, 2001; 74:596–602.

3: The Mediterranean Method for Weight Loss

Álvarez-Pérez, J.; et al. PREDIMED Study investigators: influence of a Mediterranean dietary pattern on body fat distribution: results of the PREDIMED-Canarias Intervention Randomized Trial. *Journal of the American College of Nutrition*, 2016, Aug.; 35(6):568–80.

Bertoli, S.A.; Spadafranca, A.A.; et al. Adherence to the Mediterranean diet is inversely related to binge eating disorder in patients seeking a weight loss program. *Clinical Nutrition*, 2015; 34:107–14.

Huo, R.; Du, T.; et al. Effects of Mediterranean style diet on glycemic control, weight loss, and cardiovascular risk factors among type 2 diabetes individuals: a meta-analysis. *European Journal of Clinical Nutrition*, 2015; 69:1200–208.

Lombardo, M.; Bellia, A.; et al. Morning meal more efficient for fat loss in a 3-month lifestyle intervention. *Journal of the American College of Nutrition*, 2014; 33(3):198–205.

Mancini, J.G.; et al. Systematic review of the Mediterranean diet for long-term weight loss. *American Journal of Medicine*, 2016; 129:407–15.

4: The Mediterranean Method for Heart Health

De Lorgeril, M.; et al. Mediterranean alpha-linolenic acid-rich diet in secondary prevention of coronary heart disease. *Lancet*, 1994; 343:1454–59.

De Lorgeril, M.; Salen, P.; et al. Mediterranean diet, traditional risk factors, and the rate of complications after myocardial infarction—final report of the Lyon Diet Heart Study. *Circulation*, 1999; 99:779–85.

Estruch, R.; et al. For the PREDIMED Study investigators: primary prevention of cardiovascular disease with a Mediterranean diet. *New England Journal of Medicine*, 2018; 378(25):2441–42.

Forrester, J.S. Role of plaque rupture in acute coronary syndromes. *American Journal of Cardiology*, 2000; 86:15–23.

Hu, F.B.; Stampfer, J.M.; et al. Frequent nut consumption and risk of coronary heart disease in women. *BMJ*, 1998; 17:1341–45.

Kris-Etherton, P.M.; Ahao, G.; et al. The effects of nuts on coronary heart disease risk. *Nutrition Reviews*, 2001; 59:103–11.

Masley, S.C.; et al. Efficacy of exercise and diet to modify markers of fitness and wellness. *Alternative Therapies in Health and Medicine*, 2008; 14:24–29.

Masley, S.C. Dietary therapy for preventing and treating coronary artery disease. *American Family Physician*, 1998; 57:1299–306.

Nordmann, A.J.; et al. Meta-analysis comparing Mediterranean to low-fat diets for modification of cardiovascular risk factors. *American Journal of Medicine*, 2011; 124:841–51.

Rimm, E.B.; Ellison, R.C. Alcohol in the Mediterranean diet. *American Journal of Clinical Nutrition*, 1995; 61:1378–82.

Smith, S.C. Need for a paradigm shift: the importance of risk factor reduction therapy in treating patients with cardiovascular disease. *American Journal of Cardiology*, 1998; 82:10–13.

Turati, F.; et al. Glycemic load and coronary heart disease in a Mediterranean population: the EPIC Greek cohort study. *Nutrition, Metabolism & Cardiovascular Diseases*, 2015; 25:336e342.

Yusuf, S.; Hawken, S.; et al. Effect of potentially modifiable risk factors associated with myocardial infarction in 52 countries (the INTERHEART study). *Lancet*, 2004; 364:937–52.

5: The Mediterranean Method for a Better Brain

Alonso-Alonso, M. Cocoa flavanols and cognition: regaining chocolate in old age? *American Journal of Clinical Nutrition*, 2015; 101:423–24.

Baker, L.D.; et al. Insulin resistance is associated with Alzheimer-like reductions in regional cerebral glucose metabolism for cognitively normal adults with pre-diabetes or early type 2 diabetes. *Archives of Neurology*, 2011; 68:51–57.

Berr, C.; Portet, F.; et al. Olive oil and cognition: results from the three-city study. *Dementia and Geriatric Cognitive Disorders*, 2009, Oct.; 28(4): 357–64. doi: 10.1159/000253483.

Buettner, Dan. The island where people forget to die. *New York Times Magazine*, October 28, 2012. www.nytimes.com/2012/10/28/magazine/the-island-where-people-forget-to-die.html.

Crane, P.K.; et al. Glucose levels and risk of dementia. *New England Journal of Medicine*, 2013; 369:540–48.

Haller, S.; et al. Acute caffeine administration effect on brain activation patterns in mild cognitive impairment. *Journal of Alzheimer's Disease*, 2014; 41:101–12.

Martinez-Lapiscina, E.H.; Clavero, P.; et al. Mediterranean diet improves cognition: the

PREEDIMED-NAVARRA randomized trial. *Journal of Neurological Neurosurgical Psychiatry*, 2013; 84:1318–25.

Masley, S.C. Lifestyle approaches to prevent and manage cognitive impairment. *Primary Care Reports*, February 2018;24(2).

Masley, S.C.; Masley, L.V.; et al. Cardiovascular bio-markers and carotid IMT scores as predictors of cognitive function. *Journal of the American College of Nutrition*, 2014; 33:63–69.

Masley, S.C.; Roetzheim, R.; et al. Aerobic exercise enhances cognitive flexibility. *Journal of Clinical Psychology*, 2009; 16:186–93.

Masley, S.C.; Roetzheim, R.; et al. Lifestyle markers predict cognitive function. *Journal of the American College of Nutrition*, 2017; 36:617–23.

Mastroiacovo, D.; et al. Cocoa flavanol consumption improves cognitive function, blood pressure control, and metabolic profile in elderly subjects: the Cocoa, Cognition, and Aging (CoCoA) Study—a randomized controlled trial. *American Journal of Clinical Nutrition*, 2015; 101:538–48.

Matsumoto, C.; et al. Chocolate consumption and risk of diabetes mellitus in the Physicians' Health Study. *American Journal of Clinical Nutrition*, 2015; 101:362–67.

Matsuzaki, T.; et al. Insulin resistance is associated with the pathology of Alzheimer's disease. *Neurology*, 2010; 75:764–70.

Morris, M.C. The role of nutrition in Alzheimer's disease: epidemiological evidence. *European Journal of Neurology*, 2009, Sept.; 16(Suppl. 1):1–7.

Morris, M.C.; et al. Fish consumption and cognitive decline with age in a large community study. *Archives of Neurology*, 2005; 62:1849–53.

Ngandu, T.; et al. A 2 year multidomain intervention of diet, exercise, cognitive training, and vascular risk monitoring versus control to prevent cognitive decline in at-risk elderly people (FINGER): a randomised control panel. *Lancet*, 2015; 385:2255–63.

Qin, B.; et al. Fish intake is associated with slower cognitive decline in Chinese older adults. *Journal of Nutrition*, 2014; 144:1579–85.

Ronnemaa, E.; et al. Impaired insulin secretion increases the risk of Alzheimer disease. *Neurology*, 2008; 71:1065–71.

Schilling, M.A. Unraveling Alzheimer's: making sense of the relationship between diabetes and Alzheimer's disease. *Journal of Alzheimer's Disease*, 2016; 51:961–77.

Tosto, G.; Bird, T.D.; et al. National Institute on Aging Late-Onset Alzheimer Disease/National Cell Repository for Alzheimer Disease (NIA-LOAD/NCRAD) Family Study Group. *JAMA Neurology*, 2016, Oct. 1; 73(10):1231–37. doi: 10.1001/jamaneurol.2016.2539.

Willette, A.A.; et al. Association of insulin resistance with cerebral glucose uptake in late middle-aged adults at risk for Alzheimer disease. *JAMA Neurology*, 2015; 72:1013–20.

Wu, L.; Sun, D.; et al. Coffee intake and the incident risk of cognitive disorders: a dose-response meta-analysis of nine prospective cohort studies. *Clinical Nutrition*, 2016; 36:730–36.

Ye, X.; Scott, T.; et al. Mediterranean diet, healthy eating index-2005, and cognitive function in middle-aged and older Puerto Rican adults. *Journal of the Academy of Nutrition and Dietetics*, 2013; 113:276–81.

6: The Mediterranean Method for a Healthy Gut

Borzì, A.M.; Biondi, A.; et al. Olive oil effects on colorectal cancer. *Nutrients*, 2019; 1(1):32.

Hiel, S.; Bindels, L.B.; et al. Effects of a diet based on inulin-rich vegetables on gut health and nutritional behavior in healthy humans. *American Journal of Clinical Nutrition*, 2019; 109:1683–95.

Ryan, C.R.; Itsiopoulos, C.; et al. The Mediterranean diet improves hepatic steatosis and insulin sensitivity in individuals with non-alcoholic fatty liver disease. *Journal of Hepatology*, 2013; 59:138–43.

Schiattarella, G.G.; Sannino, A.; et al. Gut microbe-generated metabolite trimethylamine-N-oxide as cardiovascular risk biomarker: a systematic review and dose-response meta-analysis. *European Heart Journal*, 2017, Oct. 14; 38(39):2948–56.

7: The Mediterranean Method for Longevity

Ansberry, Clare. The advantages and limitations of living to 100. *Wall Street Journal*, May 21, 2019.

Arranz, S.; Chiva-Blanch, G.; et al. Wine, beer, alcohol and polyphenols on cardiovascular disease and cancer. *Nutrients*, 2012, July; 4(7):759–81.

Bagnardi, V.l.; Randi, G.; et al. Alcohol consumption and lung cancer risk in the Environment and Genetics in Lung Cancer Etiology (EAGLE) study. *American Journal of Epidemiology*, 2010, Jan. 1; 171(1):36–44.

Berger, K.; Ajani, U.A.; et al. Light-to-moderate alcohol consumption and the risk of stroke among U.S. male physicians. *New England Journal of Medicine*, 1999, Nov. 18; 341(21):1557–64.

Borzì, A.M.; Biondi, A.; et al. Olive oil effects on colorectal cancer. *Nutrients*, 2019, Jan.; 11(1):32.

Boston University. The New England Centenarian Study. www.bumc.bu.edu/centenarian/

Bravi, F.; et al. Mediterranean diet and bladder cancer risk in Italy. *Nutrients*, 2018; 19:1061.

Central Intelligence Agency. https://www.cia.gov/library/publications/the-world-factbook/rankorder/2102rank.html

CEO World Magazine. https://ceoworld.biz/2019/02/28/countries-with-the-highest-average-life-expectancies-in-2030/

García-Calzón, S.; Martínez-González, M.A.; et al. Pro12Ala polymorphism of the PPARγ2 gene interacts with a Mediterranean diet to prevent telomere shortening in the PREDIMED-NAVARRA randomized trial. *Circulation: Cardiovascular Genetics*, 2015, Feb.; 8(1):91–99.

Giacosaa, A.; Baralec, R.; et al. Cancer prevention in Europe: the Mediterranean diet as a protective choice. *European Journal of Cancer Prevention*, 2013; 22:90–95.

Grønbaek, M.; Becker, U.; et al. Population based cohort study of the association between alcohol intake and cancer of the upper digestive tract. *BMJ*, 1998; 317:844–47.

Holahan, C.J.; et al. Wine consumption and 20-year mortality among late life moderate drinkers. *Annals of Internal Medicine*, 2000; 133:411–19.

Huo, R.; Du, T.; et al. Effects of Mediterranean-style diet on glycemic control, weight loss and cardiovascular risk factors among type 2 diabetes individuals: a meta-analysis. *European Journal of Clinical Nutrition*, 2015; 69:1200–208.

Ibarrola-Jurado, N.; et al. Cross-sectional assessment of nut consumption and obesity, metabolic syndrome, and other cardiometabolic risk factors: The PREDIMED Study. *PLOS ONE*, 2013; 8:e57367.

Jankovic, N.; Geelen, A.; et al. Adherence to a healthy diet according to the World Health Organization guidelines and all-cause mortality in elderly adults from Europe and the United States. *American Journal of Epidemiology*, 2014, Nov. 15; 180(10):978–88.

Klatsky, A.L.; Armstrong, M.A.; et al. Alcohol and mortality. *Annals of Internal Medicine*, 1992, Oct. 15; 117(8):646–54.

Papa, N.P.; MacInnis, R.J.; et al. Total and beverage-specific alcohol intake and the risk of aggressive prostate cancer: a case-control study. *Prostate Cancer and Prostatic Diseases*, 2017, Sept.; 20(3):305–10.

Ratjen, I.; Schafmayer, C.; et al. Postdiagnostic Mediterranean and healthy Nordic dietary patterns are inversely associated with all-cause mortality in long-term colorectal cancer survivors. *Journal of Nutrition*, 2017, Apr.; 147(4):636–44.

Schwingshackl, L.; Schwedhelm, C.; et al. Adherence to Mediterranean diet and risk of cancer: an updated systematic review and meta-analysis. *Nutrients*, 2017, Oct.; 9(10):1063. PMID: 28954418.

Shammas, Masood A. Telomeres, lifestyle, cancer, and aging: current opinion in clinical nutrition and metabolic care. *Current Opinion in Clinical Nutrition and Metabolic Care*, 2011; 14:28–34. doi:10.1097/MCO.0b013e32834121b1.

Thun, M.J.; Peto, R.; et al. Alcohol consumption and mortality among middle-aged and elderly U.S. adults. *New England Journal of Medicine*, 1997, Dec. 11; 337(24):1705–14.

Willcox, D.C.; Scapagnini, G.; et al. Healthy aging diets other than the Mediterranean: a focus on the Okinawan diet. *Mechanisms of Ageing and Development*, 2014; 136:148–62.

World Population Review. http://worldpopulation review.com/countries/life-expectancy/

8: Bringing the Mediterranean Diet Home

Centers for Disease Control. https://www.cdc.gov/media/releases/2018/p0118-smoking-rates-declining.html

European Union. https://publications.europa.eu/en/publication-detail/-/publication/2f01a3d1-0af2-11e8-966a-01aa75ed71a1/language-en

Lombardo, M.; Bellia, A.; et al. Morning meal more efficient for fat loss in a 3-month lifestyle intervention. *Journal of the American College of Nutrition*, 2014; 33(3):198–205.

Vasto, S.; Buscemi, S.; et al. Mediterranean diet and healthy ageing: a Sicilian perspective. *Gerontology*, 2014; 60(6):508–18.

Acknowledgments

Numerous people have made this book possible, and I am deeply grateful for their assistance. Many thanks to my literary agents, Celeste Fine and John Mass—they have been inspirational in guiding me throughout the production of this book.

I owe a special thanks to Becky Cabaza, a talented and experienced writer, who helped me organize this material and convert complex medical information into an easy-to-read and lively discussion. I also feel fortunate to have worked with my executive editor at Harmony Books, Marnie Cochran, who has provided excellent guidance to ensure that this book provides a powerful and important message and that the recipes are practical and user friendly.

I am grateful to Karen Roth and Rachelle Benzarti, the medical library staff at Morton Plant Hospital in Clearwater, Florida, for helping me to research thousands of scientific articles, which were seminal for the writing of this book. I was fortunate to have joined the Institute of Functional Medicine at its inception, and have benefited from their medical education programs over the last twenty-five years.

Several medical colleagues scheduled interviews with me to discuss material related to this book. I'd especially like to thank JJ Virgin, David Perlmutter MD, Stephen Sinatra, MD, Sara Gottfried, MD, Anna Cabeca, DO, and Alan Christianson, NMD.

Over the last twenty-five years, my research has been supported by numerous organizations, including the American College of Nutrition, the American Heart Association, Morton Plant Hospital, and Group Health Cooperative; as well as collaboration from medical colleagues including Richard Roetzheim, MD, Douglas Schocken, MD, Tom Gualtieri, MD, and Lucas Masley, BS. I am grateful for their time and consideration.

I have also been assisted by a group who tested and reviewed many of the recipes in this book. Foremost is my wife, Nicole, who provided helpful hints regarding many of the recipes. I would also like to thank Marcos Masley, Brooke Masley, Peggy Masley, and Michelle and Gary Crosby for their feedback and help in cooking and tasting various recipes.

I would like to extend a special thanks to my patients. Not only have they agreed to participate in studies at my clinic, providing me with invaluable data, but they have also helped me convert this technical information into everyday words that empower people along a path to being healthier, trimmer, and physiologically younger; their struggles and triumphs continue to be my inspiration. My medical team at the Masley Optimal Health Center has also been very supportive in the production of this manuscript, with special thanks to Tarin Forbes, DO, my new medical partner who has permitted me to take an extended sabbatical to travel the Mediterranean Sea, plus our staff: Angie Presby, Jen York, and Heather Franczkowski. Also, thanks to my on-line coordinator, Kim Escarraz, who has supported all my speaking, writing, and blogging activities.

Lastly, I want to extend a special thanks to my loving wife, Nicole. Not only has she aided my research, patient care, and recipe writing, but she has helped me in every aspect of my life, including providing me with love and support, even while fulfilling my dream to sail across the Mediterranean Sea.

Index

matcha green tea, 40
MCT oil, 105
meat, red. *See* red meat
Mediterranean diet
    daily featured foods, 10, 20–21, 31–41
    do's and don'ts, 23–27
    geographic regions, 18
    global adoption of, 19–20
    health benefits, 10–11
    occasional foods, 10, 19, 50–54
    weekly featured foods, 43–49
Mediterranean Method
    for a better brain, 96–109
    food pyramid, 22–23, 63
    for a healthy gut, 111–25
    for heart health, 75–94
    lifestyle component, 22
    for longevity, 127–40
    origins of, 13, 21
    overview, 13
    social component, 22
    for weight loss, 56–73
Mediterranean Method stories
    improving cognitive function, 108
    reversing heart disease, 93
    weight loss success, 71–72
memory loss, 96–109
mercury, 45, 107
metabolic syndrome, 131–33
metabolism, 69
milk protein allergy, 124
mindfulness, 69–70, 106, 143–45
multiple sclerosis, 122
multivitamins, 104, 144
Mushroom(s)
    and Marinara Sauce, Spaghetti with, 172–73
    Spinach, and Cheese, Frittata with, 166
    Wild, Omelet, Mediterranean, 164

NAFLD (non-alcoholic fatty liver disease), 120
Nicoya, Costa Rica, 20
nitrosamines, 106–7
NSAIDs, 115
nuts, 32–33, 153, 159

Oats
    Berries and Yogurt with Toasted Muesli, 165
    Berry and Apple Crumble, 225
    Hot Steel-Cut Oatmeal with Apple, Berries, and Nuts, 167
oils, 152. *See also* olive oil
Okinawa, Japan, 20, 44, 129
olive oil, 26, 33–35, 83, 136

olives, 35
Olives, Marinated Mediterranean, and Vegetables, 170
omega-3 fats, 24, 44–45, 86, 87–88, 103–4
Omelets
    Mediterranean Wild Mushroom, 164
    Spanish Tortilla, 209
Ornish program, 12, 13
oxidative stress, 100–101

pantry staples, 151–53
Pasta, 24, 41–42, 47
    Greek Lemon, Chicken, and Orzo Soup, 177
    Linguine with Frutti di Mare, 192–93
    Spaghetti with Marinara Sauce and Mushrooms, 172–73
Peaches and Berries with Muscatel Wine and Mint, 224
Pears Poached with Wine and Cinnamon, 222
Perlmutter, David, 102
Pesto, 227
physical activity, 41–42, 61. *See also* exercise
plaque rupture, 79
polyphenols, 138
Pomegranate and Black-Eyed Pea Salad, 212
portion control, 18, 24
potassium, 92
Potatoes, 52–53
    Spanish Tortilla (Omelet), 209
    Sweet, Mashed, and Port Wine Sauce, Duck with, 203
poultry, 46. *See also* Chicken; Duck; Turkey
prebiotics, 116, 118
pre-diabetes, 132
PREDIMED study, 62, 77, 99–101, 132
Pritikin plan, 13, 21
probiotics, 36–37, 48–49, 59, 119
probiotic supplements, 104, 116
processed foods, 10, 18, 25–26, 64–65, 66, 84
prostate cancer, 137
protein
    at breakfast, 67–68, 148–49
    choosing, 43–44, 66–67
    GL values, 161

red meat, 10, 18, 50–51, 84, 136
red wine, 38–39
    from Cannonau grapes, 20, 38
    GL values, 161
    health benefits, 26, 58, 138
resistant starch, 52–53
restaurant meals, 147
resveratrol, 59, 105

About the Author

STEVEN MASLEY, MD, is a physician, nutritionist, trained chef, and author. A fellow with the American Heart Association and the American College of Nutrition, he has helped thousands of patients improve their cognitive function, and prevent and reverse type II diabetes and heart disease. His clinical research focuses on the impact of lifestyle choices on brain function, heart health, and aging. Dr. Masley has published several best-selling books, including *The Better Brain Solution, The 30-Day Heart Tune-Up, Ten Years Younger, Smart Fat,* and numerous scientific articles that have appeared in *The Journal of the American College of Nutrition, Integrative Medicine, JAMA, The American Family Physician,* and *The Journal of Clinical Psychology.* His health programs have been seen on PBS, the Discovery Channel, and the *Today* show. Dr. Masley is a Clinical Professor with the University of South Florida. He lives in St. Petersburg, Florida.

www.drmasley.com
Facebook: @StevenMasley
Instagram: #stevenmasleymd

OTHER TITLES BY STEVEN MASLEY, M.D.

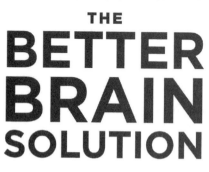

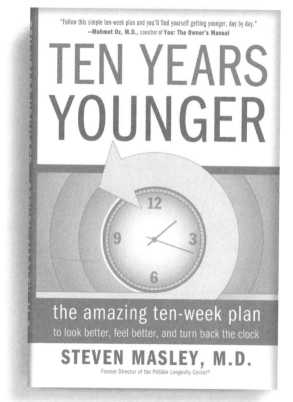

Available everywhere books are sold